SPANISH FOR HOSPITAL PERSONNEL

By

JOSEPHINE CARREÑO, M.A.

Instructor in Spanish

Holy Cross High School

Flushing, New York

DIANE LARSON, M.A.

Instructor in Spanish

Christ the King High School

Middle Village, New York

MEDICAL EXAMINATION PUBLISHING COMPANY, INC.

65-36 Fresh Meadow Lane

Flushing, N.Y. 11365

Library of Congress
Catalog Card Number

76-182582

ISBN 0-87488-722-4

January, 1974

PRINTED IN THE UNITED STATES OF AMERICA

FOREWORD

     Having taught Spanish to hospital personnel - doctors, nurses, laboratory technicians, social workers and others - for several years now, we felt that this type of handbook would be a useful tool, not only as an adjunct to teaching functional Spanish, geared toward this particular area, but also to serve as a convenient guide and easy reference for those on the hospital staff who deal with Spanish-speaking patients who have little or no knowledge of English.

     In emergency situations, a key word or expression may elicit vital information. To this end, we have also included a vocabulary germane to the services of each area covered.

     The phonetic indications will help even the least initiated in the language to pronounce understandably.

     We have aimed at maximum clarity, pertinence and conciseness in the questions and statements set forth in each section, and trust that this manual will be helpful in bridging the language barrier - that it will be an aid to more effective communication.

J. C.

D. L.

PREFACE

"The Medium is The Message" a phrase conceived by the eminent communications expert Marshall McLuhan has borne an insightful, necessary view of the hospitalized patient. Rarely has the need for communication proven more essential than in a hospital environment.

With this in mind, this book is comprised of the essential grammar and phraseology necessary for communication in Spanish within a modern hospital.

With the ever-increasing migration of Spanish-speaking people to large metropolitan areas of the United States and their subsequent requirement of medical care, knowledge of the Spanish language becomes a virtual necessity in a hospital. For a physician, taking the history is the most essential factor in the diagnosis of the patient's illness. For other members of the health care team, nurses, physical therapists, technicians and social workers communication is the key to the achievement of the comfort, treatment and rehabilitation of the patient. Most importantly, language is the only means by which a health care worker and a frightened patient can enter into a relationship of cooperation and trust so necessary to the goals of both.

This is not a grammar book, but rather a book that teaches the living language. It has a minimum of rules and a maximum of practicality. It treats everyday occurrences with a special tendency towards facets connected with hospital life. For the health-care worker faced with the task of communicating in a foreign language the authors present the fundamentals as ideas in complete sentences instead of fragmented phrases.

I wish to applaud the Misses Larsen and Carreño for their foresight and desire to help those Spanish-speaking, hospitalized patients whose needs must be understood, especially in emergencies. Furthermore, this handy guide will go far to alleviate the frustrations and indignities resulting from the lack of communication so common in the modern metropolitan hospital today.

William A. D'Angelo, M. D.
Associate Professor of Medicine
Health Sciences School
    of Medicine
State University of New York
    at Stony Brook

SPANISH FOR HOSPITAL PERSONNEL

TABLE OF CONTENTS

DEDICATED TO:

Albert

Robert

Kenneth

BBB

BASIC RULES FOR PRONUNCIATION

Spanish is pronounced as it is written.

The vowels have one, pure sound:

a (ah) as in "papa"

e (eh) as in "lemon"

i (ee) as in "reek"

o (aw) as in "raw"

u (oo) as in "ooze." NOTE: The "u" in combination with "q" is silent unless it has two dots over it, when it is pronounced like the English "w," as in "quick."

THE CONSONANTS:

b (beh) as in "bell"

c (seh) as in "cell." NOTE: The "c" before "e" or "i" has an "s" sound, as in "cinder," "cemetery." The "c" before "a," "o" or "u," has a "k" sound, as in "call," "coma," "curl."

ch (cheh) as in "chore."

d (deh) The tip of the tongue comes slightly between the front teeth, giving the sound of a hard "th," as in "this," "though."

f (eh-feh) as in "full"

g (heh) as in "her." NOTE: The "g" before "e" or "i" has an aspirate sound, as in "hem," "hill." The "g" before "a," "o" or "u," has a hard sound as in "gamble," "go," "gun."

h (ah-cheh) The "h" is always silent.

j (haw-tah) Has the sound of the English "h" in "ham."

k (kah) Rarely used except in words of foreign origin. Pronounced like the English "k" in "king."

l (eh-leh) as in "line"

ll (eh-yeh) Pronounced like the English "y," as in "your"

m (eh-meh) as in "mama"

n (eh-neh) as in "note"

ñ (eh-nyeh) Prounced like the "ny" in "canyon"

p (peh) as in "poor"

q (koo) The "q," in combination with a silent "u," as in "que" (keh), "qui" (kee), is pronounced as the English "k" in "kettle," "keen."

r (eh-reh) Pronounced with a single flip of the tongue against the upper front teeth.

rr (<u>ehr</u>-reh) Pronounced with a triple flip of the tongue against the upper front teeth. NOTE: This applies also to the single "r" when it is at the beginning of a word.

s (<u>eh</u>-seh) Soft sound of "s, " as in "sister. "

t (teh) The tongue touching the upper front teeth, gives the "t" a softer sound than the English "t"; it is closer to the sound of "th, " as in "thought. "

v (beh) Same as the Spanish "b"

w (daw-bleh-beh) Used only in words of foreign origin.   Pronounced like the <u>English</u> "w"

x (<u>eh</u>-kees) as in "exit"

y (<u>ee</u>-<u>gryeh</u>-gah) Pronounced like the "y" in "yawn"; also like the Spanish "i" (<u>ee</u>), as in the word "y" (and).

z (<u>seh</u>-tah) like the English "s" in "sad"

ACCENTUATION:

Words ending in a vowel, or in the consonants "n" or "s, " are accented on the next to the last syllable: "hombre (<u>awm</u>-breh), "agua" (<u>ah</u>-gwah).

Words ending in a consonant, except "n" or "s, " are accented on the last syllable: "señor" (seh-<u>nyawr</u>), "español" (ehs-pah-<u>nyawl</u>).

Words that do not conform to these rules carry a written accent: "café" (kah-<u>feh</u>) = "coffee"; "aquí" (ah-<u>kee</u>) = "here. "

ℰℬℰℬℰℬ

BASIC CONCEPTS

DEFINITE ARTICLE

the = el (before a singular, masculine noun): el hombre (the man)
    la (before a singular, feminine noun): la mujer (the woman)
    los (before a plural, masculine noun): los brazos (the arms)
    las (before a plural, feminine noun): las piernas (the legs)

INDEFINITE ARTICLE

a, an = un (before a singular, masculine noun): un médico (a doctor)
    una (before a singular, feminine noun): una enfermera (a nurse)

> NOTE: the plural forms of the masculine and feminine render
> the meaning of "some": unas píldoras (some pills)
> unos platos (some plates)

SUBJECT PRONOUNS

Singular	Plural
I = yo	we = nosotros
you = tú (familiar)	you = ustedes
you = usted (formal)	they = ellos (masculine)
he = él	they = ellas (feminine)
she = ella	

INTERROGATIVE ADJECTIVES AND PRONOUNS

When?	¿Cuándo? (kwahn-daw)
Where?	¿Dónde? (dawn-deh)
What?	¿Qué? (keh)
What?	¿Cuál? (kwahl) (used before the verb "ser," followed by a noun: Cuál es su nombre? (What is your name?)
Which?	¿Cuál? (when making a choice: ¿Cuál de los libros quiere? (Which book do you want?)
Which? (plural)	¿Cuáles? (kwah-lehs) ¿Cuáles de los libros quiere? (Which books do you want?)
Who? (singular)	¿Quién? (kyehn)
Who? (plural)	¿Quiénes? (kyeh-nehs)
Whose?	¿De quién? (deh kyehn)
How?	¿Cómo? (kaw-maw)
Why?	¿Por qué? (pawr-keh)
How much?	¿Cuánto? (kwahn-taw)
How many? (masculine)	¿Cuántos? (kwahn-taws)
How many? (feminine)	¿Cuántas? (kwahn-tahs)
With whom?	¿Con quién? (kawn kyehn)
For Whom?	¿Para quién? (pah-rah kyehn)
To whom?	¿A quién? (ah kyehn)

DEMONSTRATIVE PRONOUNS

	Singular		Plural
this (these)	éste (masc.)	(ehs-teh)	éstos (ehs-taws)
	ésta (fem.)	(ehs-tah)	éstas (ehs-tahs)
that (those)	ése (masc.)	(eh-seh)	ésos (eh-saws)
	ésa (fem.)	(eh-sah)	ésas (eh-sahs)
that (those)	aquél (masc.)	(ah-kehl)	aquéllos (ah-keh-yaws)
(farther away)	aquélla (fem.)	(ah-keh-yah)	aquéllas (ah-keh-yahs)

NEUTER

this -- esto: Esto no me parece bien. (This does not seem right to me.)
that -- eso: Eso no me gusta. (I don't like that.)
       aquello: Aquello me pareció mal. (That seemed bad to me.
            [Referring to something in the past.])

EXPRESSIONS OF TIME

EXPRESIONES DE TIEMPO
(ehgs-preh-syaw-nehs deh tyehm-paw)

It's 3:15
(Before the half-hour mark,
you express the hour,
plus the minutes.)

Son las tres y cuarto. (sawn lahs
   trehs ee kwahr-taw)

It's 1:35.
(After the half-hour mark,
you express the next hour,
minus the minutes.)

Son las dos menos veinte y cinco.
  (sawn lahs daws meh-naws beheen-teh
  ee seen-kaw)

What time is it?

¿Qué hora es? (keh aw-rah ehs)

It is one o'clock exactly.

Es la una en punto. (ehs lah oo-nah
   ehn poon-taw)

It is seven P.M.

Son las siete de la tarde. (sawn lahs
   syeh-teh deh lah tahr-deh)

It is eight A.M.

Son las ocho de la mañana. (sawn lahs
   aw-chaw deh lah mahn-yah-nah)

It is late.	Es tarde. (ehs <u>tahr</u>-deh)
It is early.	Es temprano. (ehs tehm-<u>prah</u>-naw)
At noontime.	A mediodía. (ah meh-dyaw-<u>dee</u>-ah)
At midnight.	A medianoche. (ah meh-dyah-<u>naw</u> cheh)
In the morning.	Por la mañana. (pawr lah mahn-<u>yah</u>-nah)
In the afternoon.	Por la tarde. (pawr lah <u>tahr</u>-deh)
In the evening.	Por la noche. (pawr lah <u>naw</u>-cheh)
Right now.	Ahora mismo. (ah-<u>aw</u>-rah <u>meez</u>-maw)
Later.	Más tarde. (mahs <u>tahr</u>-deh)
It is time for...	Es hora de... (ehs <u>aw</u>-rah deh...)
Tonight.	Esta noche. (<u>ehs</u>-tah <u>naw</u>-cheh)
Today.	Hoy. (awy)
Last night.	Anoche. (ah-<u>naw</u>-cheh)
Afterwards.	Después. (dehs-<u>pwehs</u>)
During the day.	Durante el día. (doo-<u>rahn</u>-teh ehl <u>dee</u>-ah)
Last year.	El año pasado. (ehl <u>ahn</u>-yaw pah-<u>sah</u>-daw)
Next year.	El año próximo. (ehl <u>ahn</u>-yaw <u>prawk</u>-see-maw)
The day after tomorrow.	Pasado mañana. (pah-<u>sah</u>-daw mahn-<u>yah</u>-nah)
One moment...	Un momento... (oon maw-<u>mehn</u>-taw)
Twice a day.	Dos veces al día. (daws <u>beh</u>-sehs ahl <u>dee</u>-ah)
The day before yesterday.	Anteayer. (ahn-teh-ah-<u>yehr</u>)
Every hour.	Cada hora. (<u>kah</u>-dah <u>aw</u>-rah)
How many years?	¿Cuántos años? (<u>kwahn</u>-taws <u>ahn</u>-yaws)
Two years ago...	Hace dos años que... (<u>ah</u>-seh daws <u>ahn</u>-yaws keh...)
How many times?	¿Cuántas veces? (<u>kwahn</u>-tahs <u>beh</u>-sehs)
How often?	¿Cada qué tiempo? (<u>kah</u>-dah keh <u>tyehm</u>-paw)
What month?	¿Qué mes? (keh mehs)

How long is it since...	¿Cuánto tiempo hace que... (kwahn-taw tyehm-paw ah-seh keh...)
In what year?	¿En qué año? (ehn keh ahn-yaw)
Since this morning.	Desde esta mañana. (dehz-deh ehs-tah mahn-yah-nah)

DAYS OF THE WEEK   **LOS DÍAS DE LA SEMANA**
(laws dee-ahs deh lah seh-mah-nah)

Sunday	el domingo	(ehl daw-meen-gaw)
Monday	el lunes	(ehl loo-nehs)
Tuesday	el martes	(ehl mahr-tehs)
Wednesday	el miércoles	(ehl myehr-kaw-lehs)
Thursday	el jueves	(ehl hweh-behs)
Friday	el viernes	(ehl byehr-nehs)
Saturday	el sábado	(ehl sah-bah-daw)

MONTHS OF THE YEAR   **LOS MESES DEL AÑO**
(laws meh-sehs dehl ahn-yaw)

January	enero	(eh-neh-raw)
February	febrero	(feh-breh-raw)
March	marzo	(mahr-saw)
April	abril	(ah-breel)
May	mayo	(mah-yaw)
June	junio	(hoon-yaw)
July	julio	(hool-yaw)
August	agosto	(ah-gaws-taw)
September	septiembre	(sehp-tyehm-breh)
October	octubre	(awk-too-breh)
November	noviembre	(naw-byehm-breh)
December	diciembre	(dee-syehm-breh)

THE SEASONS   **LAS ESTACIONES**
(lahs ehs-tah-syaw-nehs)

spring	la primavera	(lah pree-mah-beh-rah
summer	el verano	(ehl beh-rah-naw)
fall	el otoño	(ehl aw-tawn-yaw)
winter	el invierno	(ehl een-byehr-naw)

COLORS   **LOS COLORES**
(laws kaw-law-rehs)

black	negro	(neh-graw)
white	blanco	(blahn-kaw)
blue	azul	(ah-sool)
gold	dorado	(daw-rah-daw)
grey	gris	(grees)
green	verde	(behr-deh)
orange	naranja	(nah-rahn-hah)
pink	rosado	(raw-sah-daw)
red	rojo	(raw-haw)
yellow	amarillo	(ah-mah-ree-yaw)
blonde	rubio	(roo-byaw)

brown	moreno	(maw-reh-naw)
clear	claro	(klah-raw)
opaque	opaco	(aw-pah-kaw)
pale	pálido	(pah-lee-daw)
transparent	trasparente	(trahs-pah-rehn-teh)

NUMBERS

Ordinal numbers: In Spanish ordinal numbers are generally used only up to ten.

the first	el primero*; la primera (ehl pree-meh-raw; lah pree-meh-rah)
the second	el segundo; la segunda (ehl seh-goon-daw; lah seh-goon-dah)
the third	el tercero*; la tercera (ehl tehr-seh-raw; lah tehr-seh-rah)
the fourth	el cuarto; la cuarta (ehl kwahr-taw; lah kwahr-tah)
the fifth	el quinto; la quinta (ehl keen-taw; lah keen-tah)
the sixth	el sexto; la sexta (ehl sehgs-taw; lah sehgs-tah)
the seventh	el séptimo; la séptima (ehl sehp-tee-maw; lah sehp-tee-mah)
the eighth	el octavo; la octava (ehl awk-tah-baw; lah awk-tah-bah)
the ninth	el noveno; la novena (ehl naw-beh-naw; lah naw-beh-nah)
the tenth	el décimo; la décima (ehl deh-see-maw; lah deh-see-mah)

*Before masculine, singular nouns, the last "o" is dropped:

el primer paciente (the first patient)
el tercer médico (the third doctor)

Cardinal numbers

1.	uno*	(oo-naw)
2.	dos	(daws)
3.	tres	(trehs)
4.	cuatro	(kwah-traw)
5.	cinco	(seen-kaw)
6.	seis	(seh-ees)
7.	siete	(syeh-teh)
8.	ocho	(aw-chaw)
9.	nueve	(nweh-beh)
10.	diez	(dyehs)
11.	once	(awn-seh)
12.	doce	(daw-seh)
13.	trece	(treh-seh)
14.	catorce	(kah-tawr-seh)
15.	quince	(keen-seh)

*Drop the "o" when it precedes a masculine noun:
un médico (one doctor [or] a doctor)

It becomes "una" before a feminine noun:
una enfermera (one nurse [or] a nurse)

16.	diez y seis	(dyehs ee seh-ees)
17.	diez y siete	(dyehs ee syeh-teh)
18.	diez y ocho	(dyehs ee aw-chaw)
19.	diez y nueve	(dyehs ee nweh-beh)
20	veinte	(behyn-teh)
30.	treinta	(trehyn-tah)
40.	cuarenta	(kwah-rehn-tah)
50.	cincuenta	(seen-kwehn-tah)
60.	sesenta	(seh-sehn-tah)
70.	setenta	(seh-tehn-tah)
80.	ochenta	(aw-chehn-tah)
90.	noventa	(naw-behn-tah)
100.	ciento*	(syehn-taw)

*Becomes "cien" when used before any noun, masculine or feminine:

cien píldoras (100 pills)
cien ojos   (100 eyes)

101.	ciento uno	(syehn-taw oo-naw)
102.	ciento dos	(syehn-taw daws)
200.	doscientos	(daws syehn-taws)
300.	trescientos	(trehs syehn-taws)
400.	cuatrocientos	(kwah-traw syehn-taws)
500.	quinientos	(kee-nyehn-taws)
600.	seiscientos	(sehys syehn-taws)
700.	setecientos	(seh-teh-syehn-taws)
800.	ochocientos	(aw-chaw-syehn-taws)
900.	novecientos	(naw-beh-syehn-taws)
1000.	mil	(meel)

ℬℬℬ

GENERAL COURTESIES

GENERAL COURTESIES	CORTESÍAS GENERALES
	(kawr-teh-<u>see</u>-ahs geh-neh-<u>rah</u>-lehs)
Good morning.	¡Buenos días! (<u>bweh</u>-naws <u>dee</u>-ahs)
Good afternoon (evening).	¡Buenas tardes! (<u>bweh</u>-nahs <u>tahr</u>-dehs)
Good night.	¡Buenas noches! (<u>bweh</u>-nahs <u>naw</u>-chehs)
Good luck!	¡Buena suerte! (<u>bweh</u>-nah <u>swehr</u>-teh)
See you later.	¡Hasta luego! (<u>ahs</u>-tah <u>lweh</u>-gaw)
Until tomorrow.	¡Hasta mañana! (<u>ahs</u>-tah mahn-<u>yah</u>-nah)
Thank you very much.	¡Muchas gracias! (<u>moo</u>-chahs <u>grah</u>-syahs)
You're welcome.	¡De nada! (deh <u>nah</u>-dah)
May I help you?	¿En qué puedo servirle? (ehn keh <u>pweh</u>-daw sehr-<u>beer</u>-leh)
How are you?	¿Cómo le va? (or) ¿Cómo está usted? (<u>kaw</u>-maw leh bah. <u>kaw</u>-maw ehs-<u>tah</u> oos-<u>tehd</u>)
I am very sorry.	Lo siento mucho. (law <u>syehn</u>-taw <u>moo</u>-chaw)
I am very glad.	Me alegro mucho. (meh ah-<u>leh</u>-graw <u>moo</u>-chaw)
I am very glad to have served you.	Estoy muy contento (contenta) de haberle servido. (ehs-<u>tawy</u> mw<u>ee</u> kawn-<u>tehn</u>-taw [kawn-<u>tehn</u>-<u>tah</u>] deh ah-<u>behr</u>-leh sehr-<u>bee</u>-daw)
Have a good rest.	Tenga un buen descanso. (<u>tehn</u>-gah oon bwehn dehs-<u>kahn</u>-saw)
May everything go well.	¡Qué le vaya bien! (keh leh <u>bah</u>-yah byehn)
Would you like....?	¿Le gustaría....? (leh goos-tah-r<u>ee</u>-yah)
May I get you anything?	¿Puedo traerle algo? (<u>pweh</u>-daw trah-<u>ehr</u>-leh <u>ahl</u>-gaw)
Everything will be fine.	Todo saldrá bien. (<u>taw</u>-daw sahl-<u>drah</u> byehn)
Don't worry.	¡No se preocupe! (naw seh preh-aw-<u>koo</u>-peh)

Please!	¡Por favor! (pawr fah-<u>bawr</u>)
Of course!	¡Por supuesto! (pawr soo-<u>pwehs</u>-taw)
You're improving!	¡Está mejorándose! (ehs-<u>tah</u> meh-haw-<u>rahn</u>-daw-seh)
Can you tell me...?	¿Podría usted decirme...? (paw-<u>dree</u>-ah oos-<u>tehd</u> deh-<u>seer</u>-meh)
Exactly!	¡Exacto! (ehg-<u>sahk</u>-taw)
Yes and no.	Sí y no. (s<u>ee</u> <u>ee</u> naw)
Surely!	¡Seguramente! (seh-goo-rah-<u>mehn</u>-teh)

ℭℭℭ

THE BODY

THE BODY	EL CUERPO (ehl <u>kwehr</u>-paw)
skeleton	el esqueleto (ehl ehs-keh-<u>leh</u>-taw)
head	la cabeza (lah kah-<u>beh</u>-sah)
skull	el cráneo (ehl <u>krah</u>-neh-aw)
hair	el pelo (ehl <u>peh</u>-law)
- black	negro (<u>neh</u>-graw)
- blond	rubio (<u>roo</u>-byaw)
- chestnut	castaño (kahs-<u>tahn</u>-yaw)
- red	rojo (<u>raw</u>-haw)
- grey	gris (<u>grees</u>)
- white	blanco (<u>blahn</u>-kaw)
temples	los sienes (laws <u>syeh</u>-nehs)
brain	el cerebro (ehl seh-<u>reh</u>-braw)
face	la cara; el rostro (lah <u>kah</u>-rah; ehl <u>raws</u>-traw)
cheekbones	los pómulos (laws <u>paw</u>-moo-laws)
nape	la nuca (lah <u>noo</u>-kah)
neck	el cuello (ehl <u>kweh</u>-yaw)
Adam's apple	la nuez de la garganta (lah nwehs deh lah gahr-<u>gahn</u>-tah)
forehead	la frente (lah <u>frehn</u>-teh)
chin	la barba (lah <u>bahr</u>-bah)
cheeks	las mejillas (lahs meh-<u>hee</u>-yahs)
ears	las orejas (lahs aw-<u>reh</u>-hahs)
- inner ear	el oído (ehl aw-ee-daw)
- middle ear	el oído medio (eh<u>l</u> aw-ee-daw <u>meh</u>-dyaw)
ear lobe	el lóbulo (ehl <u>law</u>-boo-law)
eyes	los ojos (laws <u>aw</u>-haws)
pupils	las pupilas (lahs poo-<u>pee</u>-lahs)
eyelids	los párpados (laws <u>pahr</u>-pah-daws)
eyelashes	las pestañas (lahs pehs-<u>tahn</u>-yahs)
eyebrows	las cejas (lahs <u>seh</u>-hahs)

nose	la nariz (lah nah-r$\overline{ee}$s)
nostrils	las narices (lahs nah-r$\overline{ee}$-sehs)
mouth	la boca (lah baw-kah)
lips	los labios (laws lah-byaws)
- upper	superior (soo-peh-ryawr)
- lower	inferior ($\overline{ee}$n-feh-ryawr)
teeth	los dientes (laws dyehn-tehs)
- incisors	los incisivos (laws $\overline{ee}$n-s$\overline{ee}$-s$\overline{ee}$-baws)
- canines	los caninos (laws kah-n$\overline{ee}$-naws)
- molars	las muelas (lahs mweh-lahs)
throat	la garganta (lah gahr-gahn-tah)
jaw	la mandíbula (lah mahn-dee-boo-lah)
tongue	la lengua (lah lehn-gwah)
palate	el paladar (ehl pah-lah-dahr)
tonsils	las amígdalas (lahs ah-m$\overline{ee}$g-dah-lahs)
trunk	el tronco (ehl trawn-kaw)
heart	el corazón (ehl kaw-rah-sawn)
chest (breast)	el pecho (ehl peh-chaw)
aorta	la aorta (lah ah-awr-tah)
back	la espalda (lah ehs-pahl-dah)
ribs	las costillas (lahs kaws-t$\overline{ee}$-yahs)
belly	el vientre (ehl byehn-treh)
lungs	los pulmones (laws pool-maw-nehs)
bronchial tubes	los bronquios (laws brawn-kyaws)
abdomen	el abdomen (ehl ahb-daw-mehn)
stomach	el estómago (ehl ehs-taw-mah-gaw)
pancreas	el páncreas (ehl pahn-kreh-ahs)
liver	el hígado (ehl $\overline{ee}$-gah-daw)
spleen	el bazo (ehl bah-saw)
intestines	los intestinos (laws $\overline{ee}$n-tehs-t$\overline{ee}$-naws)
kidney	el riñon (ehl r$\overline{ee}$n-yawn)
bladder	la vejiga (lah beh-h$\overline{ee}$-gah)

ovary	el ovario (ehl aw-bah-ryaw)
vagina	la vagina (lah bah-hee-nah)
womb	la matriz (lah mah-trees)
waist	la cintura (lah seen-too-rah)
rectum	el recto (ehl rehk-taw)
anus	el ano (ehl ah-naw)
hip	la cadera (lah kah-deh-rah)
groin	la ingle (lah een-gleh)
arm	el brazo (ehl brah-saw)
forearm	el antebrazo (ehl ahn-teh-brah-saw)
wrist	la muñeca (lah moon-yeh-kah)
hand	la mano (lah mah-naw)
finger	el dedo (ehl deh-daw)
- thumb	el pulgar (ehl pool-gahr)
- index	el índice (ehl een-dee-seh)
- middle finger	el dedo del corazón (ehl deh-daw-dehl kaw-rah-sawn)
- ring finger	el anular (ehl ah-noo-lahr)
- pinky	el meñique (ehl mehn-yee-keh)
finger nails	las uñas (las oon-yahs)
knuckle	el nudillo (ehl noo-dee-yaw)
leg	la pierna (lah pyehr-nah)
thigh	el muslo (ehl moos-law)
knee	la rodilla (lah raw-dee-yah)
calf	la pantorilla (lah pahn-taw-ree-yah)
ankle	el tobillo (ehl taw-bee-yaw)
foot	el pie (ehl pyeh)
toes	los dedos del pie (laws deh-daws dehl pyeh)
big toe	el dedo grueso (ehl deh-daw grweh-saw)
heel	el talón (ehl tah-lawn)
cadaver	el cadáver (ehl kah-dah-behr)
bones	los huesos (laws weh-saws)
blood	la sangre (lah sahn-greh)

artery   la arteria (lah ahr-teh-ryah)

circulation   la circulación (lah seer-koo-lah-syawn)

heart valves   válvulas del corazón (bahl-boo-lahs dehl
                          kaw-rah-sawn)

glands   las glándulas (lahs glahn-doo-lahs)

joints   las articulaciones (lahs ahr-tee-koo-lah-
                          syaw-nehs)

goitre   el bocio (ehl baw-syaw)

ligaments   los ligamentos (laws lee-gah-mehn-taws)

metabolism   el metabolismo (ehl meh-tah-baw-lees-maw)

mind   la mente (lah mehn-teh)

muscles   los músculos (laws moos-koo-laws)

nerves   los nervios (laws nehr-byaws)

organs   los órganos (laws awr-gah-naws)

perspiration   el sudor (ehl soo-dawr)

pores   los poros (laws paw-raws)

pulse   el pulso (ehl pool-saw)

respiration   la respiración (lah rehs-pee-rah-syawn)

respiratory system   el sistema respiratorio (ehl sees-teh-mah
                          rehs-pee-rah-taw-ryaw)

saliva   la saliva (lah sah-lee-bah)

skin   la piel; el cutis (lah pyehl; ehl koo-tees)

tendon   el tendón (ehl tehn-dawn)

weight   el peso (ehl peh-saw)

urinary system   el sistema urinario (ehl sees-teh-mah
                          oo-ree-nah-ryaw)

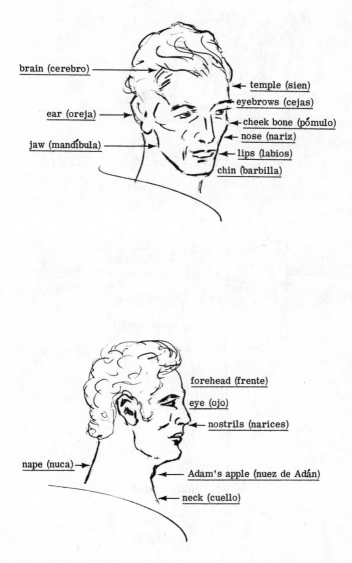

brain (cerebro)

temple (sien)

eyebrows (cejas)

ear (oreja)

cheek bone (pómulo)

nose (nariz)

jaw (mandíbula)

lips (labios)

chin (barbilla)

forehead (frente)

eye (ojo)

nostrils (narices)

nape (nuca)

Adam's apple (nuez de Adán)

neck (cuello)

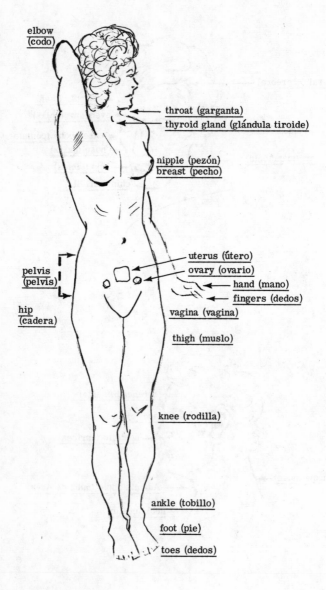

elbow
(codo)

throat (garganta)
thyroid gland (glándula tiroide)

nipple (pezón)
breast (pecho)

uterus (útero)
ovary (ovario)
hand (mano)
fingers (dedos)
vagina (vagina)

pelvis
(pelvis)

hip
(cadera)

thigh (muslo)

knee (rodilla)

ankle (tobillo)

foot (pie)

toes (dedos)

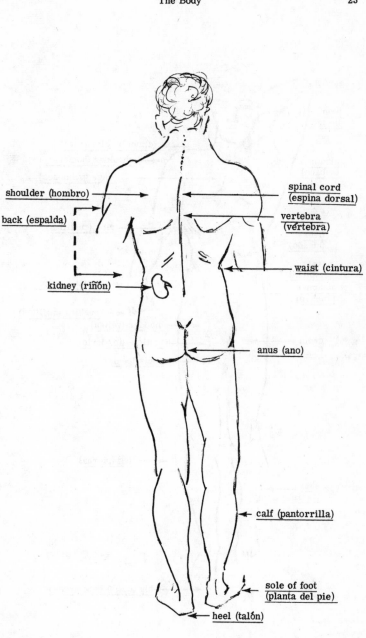

shoulder (hombro)

spinal cord (espina dorsal)

back (espalda)

vertebra (vértebra)

waist (cintura)

kidney (riñón)

anus (ano)

calf (pantorrilla)

sole of foot (planta del pie)

heel (talón)

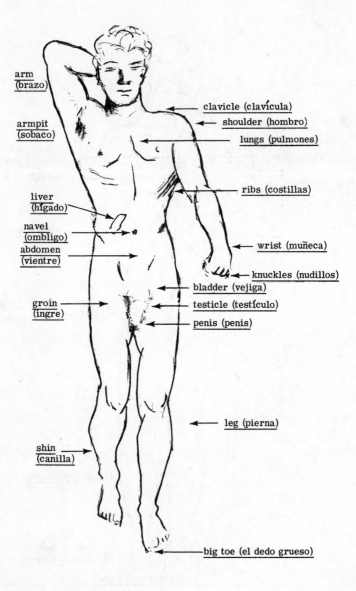

arm
(brazo)

clavicle (clavícula)

shoulder (hombro)

lungs (pulmones)

armpit
(sobaco)

ribs (costillas)

liver
(hígado)

navel
(ombligo)

abdomen
(vientre)

wrist (muñeca)

knuckles (nudillos)

bladder (vejiga)

groin
(ingre)

testicle (testículo)

penis (penis)

leg (pierna)

shin
(canilla)

big toe (el dedo grueso)

CBCB

ADMITTING OFFICE

ADMITTING OFFICE	OFICINA DE ADMISIONES (aw-fee-see-nah deh ahd-mee-syaw-nehs)
Patient's data	Datos del paciente (dah-taws dehl pah-syehn-teh)
Are you the patient?	¿Es usted el paciente? (ehs oos-tehd ehl pah-syehn-teh)
What is your name?	¿Cómo se llama? (kaw-maw seh yah-mah)
What is your address?	¿Cuál es su dirección? (kwahl ehs soo dee-rehk-syawn)
Postal zone?	¿Zona postal? (saw-nah paws-tahl)
Is this your permanent address?	¿Es ésta su dirección permanente? (ehs ehs-tah soo dee-rehk-syawn pehr-mah-nehn-teh)
Private home?	¿Casa particular? (kah-sah pahr-tee-koo-lahr)
Apartment? What number?	¿Apartamento? ¿Qué número? (ah-pahr-tah-mehn-taw. keh noo-meh-raw)
Are you the owner of your home?	¿Es usted propietario de su casa? (ehs oos-tehd praw-pyeh-tah-ryaw deh soo kah-sah)
How much is the mortgage?	¿Cuánto es la hipoteca? (kwahn-taw ehs lah ee-paw-teh-kah)
What is your telephone number?	¿Cuál es su número de teléfono? (kwahl ehs soo noo-meh-raw deh teh-leh-faw-naw)
What is your age?	¿Qué edad tiene usted? (keh eh-dahd tyeh-neh oos-tehd)
When were you born?	¿Cuándo nació usted? (kwahn-daw nah-syaw oos-tehd)
Where were you born?	¿Dónde nació usted? (dawn-deh nah-syaw oos-tehd)
How long have you lived in the U. S.?	¿Cuánto tiempo ha vivido usted en los Estados Unidos? (kwahn-taw tyehm-paw ah bee-bee-daw oos-tehd ehn laws ehs-tah-daws oo-nee-daws)

How long have you lived in N.Y.?	¿Cuánto tiempo ha vivido usted en Nueva York? (kwahn-taw tyehm-paw ah bee-bee-daw oos-tehd ehn nweh-bah yawrk)
Are you a U.S. citizen?	¿Es usted ciudadano de los Estados Unidos? (ehs oos-tehd syoo-dah-dah-naw deh laws ehs-tah-daws oo-nee-daws)
Are you single or married?	¿Es usted soltero(a) o casado(a)? (ehs oos-tehd sawl-teh-raw [sawl-teh-rah] aw kah-sah-daw [kah-sah-dah])
What is your wife's (husband's) name?	¿Cuál es el nombre de su esposa (esposo)? (kwahl ehs ehl nawm-breh deh soo ehs-paw-sah [ehs-paw-saw])
Are you a widower (widow)?	¿Es usted viudo (viuda)? (ehs oos-tehd byoo-daw [byoo-dah])
Are you divorced?	¿Es usted divorciado (divorciada)? (ehs oos-tehd dee-bawr-syah-daw [dee-bawr-syah-dah])
Are you separated? (from your wife)	¿Es usted separado de su mujer? (ehs oos-tehd seh-pah-rah-daw deh soo moo-hehr)
Are you separated? (from your husband)	¿Es usted separada de su marido? (ehs oos-tehd seh-pah-rah-dah deh soo mah-ree-daw)
What is the complete name of your father? Your mother?	¿Cuál es el nombre completo de su padre? ¿De su madre? (kwahl ehs ehl nawm-breh kawn-pleh-taw deh soo pah-dreh. deh soo-mah-dreh)
Are your parents living or dead?	¿Sus padres están vivos o muertos? (soos pah-drehs ehs-tahn bee-baws aw mwehr-taws)
Where were your parents born?	¿Dónde nacieron sus padres? (dawn-deh nah-syeh-rawn soos pah-drehs)
What is your religion?	¿Cuál es su religión? (kwahl ehs soo reh-lee-hyawn)
Protestant, Jewish, Catholic?	¿Protestante, judía, católica? (praw-tehs-tahn-teh, hoo-dee-ah, kah-taw-lee-kah)
What type of work do you do?	¿Qué clase de trabajo hace usted? (keh klah-seh deh trah-bah-haw ah-seh oos-tehd)
What is your social security number?	¿Cuál es su número de seguro social? (kwahl ehs soo noo-meh-raw deh seh-goo-raw saw-syahl)

What is the name of the company in which you work?	¿ Cuál es el nombre de la compañía con que trabaja usted? (kwahl ehs ehl <u>nawm</u>-breh deh lah kawm-pah-<u>nyee</u>-ah kawn keh trah-<u>bah</u>-hah oos-<u>tehd</u>)
What is the address of the company?	¿Cuál es la dirección de la compañía? (kwahl ehs lah <u>dee</u>-rehk-<u>syawn</u> deh lah kawm-pah-<u>nyee</u>-ah)
What is the name of your employer?	¿Cuál es el nombre de su jefe? (kwahl ehs ehl <u>nawm</u>-breh deh soo <u>heh</u>-feh)
How much do you earn per week?	¿Cuánto gana usted por semana? (<u>kwahn</u>-taw <u>gah</u>-nah oos-<u>tehd</u> pawr seh-<u>mah</u>-nah)
Do you have a savings account in any bank?	¿Tiene usted cuenta de ahorros con algún banco? (<u>tyeh</u>-neh oos-<u>tehd</u> <u>kwehn</u>-tah deh ah-<u>aw</u>-raws kawn ahl-<u>goon</u> <u>bahn</u>-kaw)
Do you receive welfare aid?	¿Recibe usted ayuda del departamento de ayuda social? (reh-<u>see</u>-beh oos-<u>tehd</u> ah-<u>yoo</u>-dah dehl deh-pahr-tah-<u>mehn</u>-taw deh ah-<u>yoo</u>-dah saw-<u>syahl</u>)
Do you receive any retirement pension?	¿Recibe usted pensión de retiro? (reh-<u>see</u>-beh oos-<u>tehd</u> pehn-<u>syawn</u> deh reh-<u>tee</u>-raw)
Do you need financial aid?	¿Necesita usted ayuda financiera? (neh-seh-<u>see</u>-tah ah-<u>yoo</u>-dah <u>fee</u>-nahn-<u>syeh</u>-rah)
What is the name of your closest relative or friend?	¿Cuál es el nombre de su familiar o amigo más cercano? (kwahl ehs ehl <u>nawm</u>-breh deh soo fah-<u>meel</u>-yahr aw ah-<u>mee</u>-gaw mahs sehr-<u>kah</u>-naw)
In case of emergency may we notify him (her)?	En caso de emergencia, ¿podemos notificar a esta persona? (ehn <u>kah</u>-saw deh eh-mehr-<u>hehn</u>-syah paw-<u>deh</u>-maws naw-<u>tee</u>-<u>fee</u>-<u>kahr</u> ah ehs-<u>tah</u> pehr-<u>saw</u>-nah)
What are his address and telephone number?	¿Cuáles son su dirección y su número de teléfono? (<u>kwah</u>-lehs sawn soo <u>dee</u>-rehk-<u>syawn</u> <u>ee</u> soo <u>noo</u>-meh-raw deh teh-<u>leh</u>-<u>faw</u>-naw)
What is the name of your insurance company?	¿Cuál es el nombre de su compañía de seguros? (kwahl ehs ehl <u>nawm</u>-breh deh soo kawm-pah-<u>nyee</u>-ah deh seh-<u>goo</u>-raws)

Do you have Blue Shield, Blue Cross; any other?	¿Tiene usted Escudo Azul, Cruz Azul; alguna otra? (tyeh-neh oos-tehd ehs-koo-daw ah-sool, kroos ah-sool; ahl-goo-nah,aw-trah)
What is your policy number?	¿Cuál es el número de su póliza? (kwahl ehs ehl noo-meh-raw deh soo paw-lee-sah)
Have you been in this hospital before? When?	¿Ha estado usted en este hospital antes? ¿Cuándo? (ah ehs-tah-daw oos-tehd ehn ehs-teh aws-pee-tahl ahn-tehs. kwahn-daw)
Have you been in any other hospital?	¿Ha estado usted en cualquier otro hospital? (ah ehs-tah-daw oos-tehd ehn kwahl-kyehr aw-traw aws-pee-tahl)
Which one? For how long? When?	¿Cuál? ¿Por cuánto tiempo? ¿Cuándo? (kwahl. pawr kwahn-taw tyehm-paw. kwahn-daw)
Have you been under a doctor's care?	¿Ha estado usted bajo cuidado de un médico? (ah ehs-tah-daw oos-tehd bah-haw kwee-dah-daw deh oon meh-dee-kaw)
For what illness?	¿Para qué enfermedad? (pah-rah keh ehn-fehr-meh-dahd)
Do you have any valuables with you?	¿Tiene algo de valor con usted? (tyeh-neh ahl-gaw deh bah-lawr kawn oos-tehd)
What items are you bringing with you to the hospital?	¿Qué cosas lleva usted al hospital? (keh kaw-sahs yeh-bah oos-tehd ahl aws-pee-tahl)
Sign here, please.	¡Firme usted aquí, por favor! (feer-meh oos-tehd ah-kee pawr fah-bawr)
Thank you.	Gracias. (grah-syahs)

ADMITTING OFFICE Useful vocabulary	**OFICINA DE ADMISIONES** Vocabulario útil (aw-fee-see-nah deh ahd-mee-syaw-nehs. baw-kah-boo-lah-ryaw oo-teel)
address	la dirección (lah dee-rehk-syawn) el domicilio (ehl daw-mee-see-lyaw)
admit	admitir (ahd-mee-teer)
age (to be... years of age)	la edad (lah eh-dahd) tener ... años (teh-nehr ... ah-nyaws)
application	la solicitud (lah saw-lee-see-tud)

apartment	el apartamento (ehl ah-pahr-tah-<u>mehn</u>-taw)
Blue Cross	la Cruz Azul (lah kroos ah-<u>sool</u>)
Blue Shield	el Escudo Azul (ehl ehs-<u>koo</u>-daw ah-<u>sool</u>)
birth	el nacimiento (ehl nah-s<u>ee</u>-<u>myehn</u>-taw)
born (to be)	nacer (nah-<u>sehr</u>)
Catholic	católico (masculine) (kah-<u>taw</u>-l<u>ee</u>-kaw) católica (feminine) (kah-<u>taw</u>-l<u>ee</u>-kah)
children	los hijos (laws <u>ee</u>-haws)
citizen	el ciudadano (masculine) (ehl syoo-dah-<u>dah</u>-naw) la ciudadana (feminine) (lah syoo-dah-<u>dah</u>-nah)
company	la compañía (lah kawm-pah-<u>nyee</u>-ah)
consultation	la consulta (lah kawn-<u>sool</u>-tah)
daughter	la hija (lah <u>ee</u>-hah)
divorced	divorciado (masculine) (dee-bawr-<u>syah</u>-daw) divorciada (feminine) (dee-bawr-<u>syah</u>-dah)
doctor	el médico (ehl <u>meh</u>-d<u>ee</u>-kaw)
(to) earn money	ganar dinero (gah-<u>nahr</u> d<u>ee</u>-<u>neh</u>-raw)
father	el padre (ehl <u>pah</u>-dreh)
financial assistance	ayuda financiera (ah-<u>yoo</u>-dah f<u>ee</u>-nahn-<u>syeh</u>-rah)
friend	el amigo (masculine) (ehl ah-<u>mee</u>-gaw) la amiga (feminine) (lah ah-<u>mee</u>-gah)
hospital	el hospital (ehl aws-p<u>ee</u>-<u>tahl</u>)
husband	el esposo (ehl ehs-<u>paw</u>-saw) el marido (ehl mah-<u>ree</u>-daw)
insurance	el seguro (ehl seh-<u>goo</u>-raw)
insurance company	la compañía de seguros (lah kawm-pah-<u>nyee</u>-ah deh seh-<u>goo</u>-raws)
Jewish	judío (masculine) (hoo-d<u>ee</u>-yaw) judía (feminine) (hoo-d<u>ee</u>-yah)

job	el empleo (ehl ehm-<u>pleh</u>-yaw)
married	casado (masculine) (kah-<u>sah</u>-daw) casada (feminine) (kah-<u>sah</u>-dah)
medicine	la medicina (lah meh-d<u>ee</u>-<u>see</u>-nah)
mother	la madre (lah <u>mah</u>-dreh)
name	el nombre (ehl <u>nawm</u>-breh)
number	el número (ehl <u>noo</u>-meh-raw)
office	la oficina (lah aw-f<u>ee</u>-<u>see</u>-nah)
operation	la operación (lah aw-pehr-ah-<u>syawn</u>)
patient	el paciente (masculine) (ehl pah-<u>syehn</u>- teh) la paciente (feminine) (lah pah-<u>syehn</u>- teh)
place	el lugar (ehl loo-<u>gahr</u>) el sitio (ehl <u>see</u>-tyaw)
policy	la póliza (lah <u>paw</u>-l<u>ee</u>-sah)
Protestant	protestante (praw-tehs-<u>tahn</u>-teh)
relative	el pariente (masculine) (ehl pah-<u>ryehn</u>- teh) la pariente (feminine) (lah pah-<u>ryehn</u>- teh)
religion	la religión (lah reh-l<u>ee</u>-<u>hyawn</u>)
(to) sign	firmar (f<u>ee</u>r-<u>mahr</u>)
single (unmarried)	soltero (masculine) (sawl-<u>teh</u>-raw) soltera (feminine) (sawl-<u>teh</u>-rah)
social security	el seguro social (ehl seh-<u>goo</u>-raw saw <u>syahl</u>)
son	el hijo (ehl <u>ee</u>-haw)
telephone	el teléfono (ehl teh-<u>leh</u>-faw-naw)
United States	los Estados Unidos (laws ehs-<u>tah</u>-daws oo-n<u>ee</u>-daws)
widow	la viuda (lah <u>byoo</u>-dah)
widower	el viudo (ehl <u>byoo</u>-daw)

𝒞𝒱𝒞

EMERGENCY WARD

EMERGENCY WARD	LA SALA DE EMERGENCIA (lah sah-lah deh eh-mehr-hehn-syah)
What happened to you?	¿Qué le pasó? (keh leh pah-saw)
Did you have an accident?	¿Tuvo un accidente? (too-baw oon ahk-see-dehn-teh)
Is this person related to you or is he (she) a friend?	¿Es esta persona pariente suyo (suya), o un amigo (una amiga)? (ehs ehs-tah pehr-saw-nah pah-ryehn-teh soo-yaw [soo-yah] aw oon ah-mee-gaw [oo-nah ah-mee-gah])
Were you unconscious, or did you faint?	¿Estuvo usted inconsciente, o se desmayó? (ehs-too-baw oos-tehd een-kawn-syehn-teh aw seh dehs-mah-yaw)
How long were you unconscious?	¿Por cuánto tiempo estuvo usted inconsciente? (pawr kwahn-taw tyehm-paw ehs-too-baw oos-tehd een-kawn-syehn-teh)
I am going to give you an injection to relieve the pain.	Le voy a dar una inyección para aliviar el dolor. (leh bawy ah dahr oo-nah een-yehk-syawn pah-rah ah-lee-byahr ehl daw-lawr)
Don't move!	¡No se mueva! (naw seh mweh-bah)
You are in a state of shock.	Usted está en un estado de postración nerviosa. (oos-tehd ehs-tah ehn oon ehs-tah-daw deh paws-trah-syawn nehr-byaw-sah)
You will have to remain in the hospital until we have completed various tests.	Tiene que quedarse en el hospital hasta que completemos varios exámenes. (tyeh-neh keh keh-dahr-seh ehn ehl aws-pee-tahl ahs-tah keh kawm-pleh-tah-maws bah-ryaws ehgs-ah-meh-nehs)
What is your name?	¿Cuál es su nombre? (kwahl ehs soo nawm-breh)
What is your address?	¿Cuál es su dirección? (kwahl ehs soo dee-rehk-syawn)
What is your telephone number?	¿Cuál es su número de teléfono? (kwahl ehs soo noo-meh-raw deh teh-leh-faw-naw)
What is the name of your closest relative or friend?	¿Cuál es el nombre de su pariente o amigo más cercano? (kwahl ehs ehl nawm-breh deh soo pah-ryehn-teh aw ah-mee-gaw mahs sehr-kah-naw)

What is his (her) address and telephone number?	¿Cuál es su dirección y su número de teléfono? (kwahl ehs soo dēē-rehk-syawn ēē soo noo-meh-raw deh teh-leh-faw-naw)
What is your social security number?	¿Cuál es su número de seguro social? (kwahl ehs soo noo-meh-raw deh seh-goo-raw saw-syahl)
What is your age?	¿Cuál es su edad? (kwahl ehs soo eh-dahd)
Date of birth?	¿La fecha de nacimiento? (lah feh-chah deh nah-sēē-myehn-taw)
Where were you born?	¿Dónde nació usted? (dawn-deh nah-syaw oos-tehd)
Are you a citizen of the U. S. ?	¿Es usted ciudadano (ciudadana) de los Estados Unidos? (ehs oos-tehd syoo-dah-dah naw [syoo-dah-dah-nah] deh laws ehs-tah-daws oo-nēē-daws)
Are you married?	¿Es usted casado (casada)? (ehs oos-tehd kah-sah-daw [kah-sah-dah])
- Single?	¿Soltero (soltera)? (sawl-teh-raw [sawl-teh-rah])
- Separated?	¿Separado (separada)? (seh-pah-rah-daw [seh-pah-rah-dah])
- Divorced?	¿Divorciado (divorciada)? (dēē-bawr-syah-daw [dēē-bawr-syah-dah])
What is your religion?	¿Cuál es su religión? (kwahl ehs soo reh-lēē-hyawn)
Do you have children? How many?	¿Tiene hijos? ¿Cuántos? (tyeh-neh ēē-haws. kwahn-taws)
Where do you work?	¿Dónde trabaja usted? (dawn-deh trah-bah-hah oos-tehd)
Name of company? Address?	¿El nombre de la compañía? ¿La dirección? (ehl nawm-breh deh lah kawm-pah nyēē-ah. lah dee-rehk-syawn)
How long have you worked there?	¿Cuánto tiempo hace que trabaja allí? (kwahn-taw tyehm-paw ah-seh keh trah-bah-hah ah-yēē)
Do you have insurance?	¿Tiene usted seguros? (tyeh-neh oos-tehd seh-goo-raws)
What is your policy number?	¿Cuál es el número de la póliza? (kwahl ehs ehl noo-meh-raw deh lah paw-lēē-sah)

Let me see your card, please.	¡Déjeme ver su tarjeta, por favor! (deh-heh-meh behr soo tahr-heh-tah pawr fah-bawr)
What are your symptoms?	¿Cuáles son sus síntomas? (kwah-lehs sawn soos seen-taw-mahs)
How long have you had these symptoms?	¿Cuánto tiempo hace que sufre estos síntomas? (kwahn-taw tyehm-paw ah-seh keh soo-freh ehs-taws seen-taw-mahs)
Have you been treated for this illness before?	¿Ha sido tratado jamás para estos síntomas? (ah see-daw trah-tah-daw hah-mahs pah-rah ehs-taws seen-taw-mahs)
By whom?	¿Por quién? (pawr kyehn)
At what hospital?	¿En qué hospital? (ehn keh aws-pee-tal)
You will have to wait until the doctor can see you.	Tiene que esperar hasta que el médico pueda verle. (tyeh-neh keh ehs-peh-rahr ahs-tah keh ehl meh-dee-kaw pweh-dah behr-leh)
EMERGENCY WARD	LA SALA DE EMERGENCIA (lah sah-lah deh eh-mehr-hehn-syah)
Useful Vocabulary	Vocabulario Útil (baw-kah-boo-lah-ryaw oo-teel)
accident	el accidente (ehl ahk-see-dehn-teh)
address	la dirección (lah dee-rehk-syawn)
age	la edad (lah eh-dahd)
appointment	la cita (lah see-tah)
(to) assist	ayudar (ah-yoo-dahr)
birth	el nacimiento (ehl nah-see-myehn-taw)
(to) bleed	sangrar (sahn-grahr)
blood	la sangre (lah sahn-greh)
Blue Cross	la Cruz Azul (lah kroos ah-sool)
Blue Shield	el Escudo Azul (ehl ehs-koo-daw ah-sool)
body	el cuerpo (ehl kwehr-paw)
bone	el hueso (ehl weh-saw)
(to be) born	nacer (nah-sehr)
(to) break	romper (rawm-pehr)

broken	roto (<u>raw</u>-taw)
(to) call	llamar (yah-<u>mahr</u>)
Catholic	Católico (masculine) (kah-taw-<u>lee</u>-kaw) Católica (feminine) (kah-taw-<u>lee</u>-kah)
child	niño (masculine) (<u>neen</u>-yaw) niña (feminine) (<u>neen</u>-yah)
children	niños (mixed masculine and feminine) (<u>neen</u>-yaws) hijos (sons and daughters) (<u>ee</u>-haws)
citizen of the U. S.	ciudadano (masculine) de los Estados Unidos (syoo-dah-dah-naw deh laws ehs-<u>tah</u>-daws oo-<u>nee</u>-daws) ciudadana (feminine) (syoo-dah-<u>dah</u>-nah)
company	la compañía (lah kawm-pah-ny<u>ee</u>-ah)
date	la fecha (lah <u>feh</u>-chah)
(to) die	morir (maw-<u>reer</u>)
dead	muerto (<u>mwehr</u>-taw) (masculine) muerta (<u>mwehr</u>-tah) (feminine)
disease	la enfermedad (lah ehn-fehr-meh-<u>dahd</u>)
divorced	divorciado (masculine) (d<u>ee</u>-bawr-<u>syah</u>-daw) divorciada (feminine) (d<u>ee</u>-bawr-<u>syah</u>-dah)
doctor	el médico (ehl <u>meh</u>-d<u>ee</u>-kaw)
(to) earn	ganar (gah-<u>nahr</u>)
emergency	emergencia (eh-mehr-<u>hehn</u>-syah)
employer	el jefe (ehl <u>heh</u>-feh)
(to) faint	desmayarse (dehs-mah-<u>yahr</u>-seh)
friend	el amigo (masculine) (ehl ah-<u>mee</u>-gaw) la amiga (feminine) (lah ah-<u>mee</u>-gah)
heart attack	ataque de corazón (ah-<u>tah</u>-keh deh kaw-rah-<u>sawn</u>)
(to) help	ayudar (ah-yoo-<u>dahr</u>)
hospital	el hospital (ehl aws-p<u>ee</u>-<u>tahl</u>)
(to) hurt, pain	doler (daw-<u>lehr</u>)

injection   la inyección (lah een-yehk-syawn)

injury   la lesión (lah leh-syawn)

insurance   el seguro (ehl seh-goo-raw)

job   el empleo (ehl ehm-pleh-yaw)

Jewish   judío (masculine) (hoo-dee-yaw)
                          judía (feminine) (hoo-dee-yah)

lie down   acuéstese (ah-kwehs-teh-seh)

married   casado (masculine) (kah-sah-daw)
                          casada (feminine) (kah-sah-dah)

medicine   la medicina (lah meh-dee-see-nah)

(to) move   moverse (maw-behr-seh)

name   el nombre (ehl nawm-breh)

number   el número (ehl noo-meh-raw)

pain   el dolor (ehl daw-lawr)

pill   la píldora (lah peel-daw-rah)

policy   la póliza (lah paw-lee-sah)

pregnant   embarazada (ehm-bah-rah-sah-dah)

relative   el (la) pariente (ehl [lah] pah-ryehn-
                              teh)

(to) relieve   aliviar (ah-lee-byahr)

religion   la religión (lah reh-lee-hyawn)

(to) remain, stay   quedarse (keh-dahr-seh)

separated   separado (masculine) (seh-pah-rah-daw)
                          separada (feminine) (seh-pah-rah-dah)

silence   el silencio (ehl see-lehn-syaw)

single   soltero (masculine) (sawl-teh-raw)
                          soltera (feminine) (sawl-teh-rah)

sit down   siéntese (syehn-teh-seh)

social security   el seguro social (ehl seh-goo-raw
                              saw-syahl)

soon   dentro de poco (dehn-traw deh paw-kaw)

sprain   la torcedura (lah tawr-seh-doo-rah)

stretcher   la camilla (lah kah-mee-yah)

symptom	el síntoma (ehl <u>seen</u>-taw-mah)
telephone number	el número de teléfono (ehl <u>noo</u>-meh-raw deh teh-<u>leh</u>-faw-naw)
test	la investigación (lah <u>een</u>-behs-<u>tee</u>-gah-<u>syawn</u>)
unconscious	inconsciente (<u>een</u>-kawn-<u>syehn</u>-teh)
United States	los Estados Unidos (laws ehs-<u>tah</u>-daws oo-<u>nee</u>-daws)
(to) wait	esperar (ehs-peh-<u>rahr</u>)
work	el trabajo (ehl trah-<u>bah</u>-haw)
(to) work	trabajar (trah-bah-<u>hahr</u>)
wound	la herida (lah eh-<u>ree</u>-dah)
wounded	herido (masculine) (eh-<u>ree</u>-daw) herida (feminine) (eh-<u>ree</u>-dah)
X-rays	los rayos equis (laws <u>rah</u>-yaws eh-<u>kees</u>)

GENERAL MEDICAL INTERVIEW

GENERAL MEDICAL INTERVIEW	ENTREVISTA MÉDICA GENERAL (ehn-treh-bee-stah meh-dee-kah heh-neh-rahl)
What seems to be the problem?	¿Cuál es su problema? (kwahl ehs soo praw-bleh-mah)
How long have you had these symptoms?	¿Cuánto tiempo hace que tiene estos síntomas? (kwahn-taw tyehm-paw ah-seh keh tyeh-neh ehs-taws seen-taw-mahs)
Have you been treated for them before?	¿Ha sido tratado por ellos antes? (ah see-daw trah-tah-daw pawr eh-yaws ahn-tehs)
By whom? For how long?	¿Por quién? ¿Por cuánto tiempo? (pawr kyehn. pawr kwahn-taw tyehm-paw)
Do you suffer from insomnia?	¿Sufre usted de insomnia? (soo-freh oos-tehd deh een-sawm-nyah)
Have you lost weight recently?	¿Ha perdido peso recientemente? (ah pehr-dee-daw peh-saw reh-syehn-teh-mehn-teh)
Have you gained weight recently?	¿Ha ganado peso recientemente? (ah gah-nah-daw peh-saw reh-syehn-teh-mehn-teh)
Do you suffer from nausea?	¿Sufre usted de náusea? (soo-freh oos-tehd deh nah-oo-seh-ah)
- dizziness?	¿vértigo? (behr-tee-gaw)
- general rundown feeling?	¿lasitud? (lah-see-tood)
- nervousness?	¿nerviosidad? (nehr-byaw-see-dahd)
Have you always been fat?	¿Ha sido siempre grueso (gruesa)? (ah see-daw syehm-pre grweh-saw [grweh-sah])
- thin?	¿flaco? (masculine) (flah-kaw) ¿flaca? (feminine) (flah-kah)
Do you have indigestion?	¿Sufre de indigestión? (soo-freh deh een-dee-hehs-tyawn)
- constipation?	¿estreñimiento? (ehs-treh-nyee-myehn-taw)
- diarrhea?	¿diarrea? (dee-ah-reh-ah)

Have you noticed any blood in your stools?	¿Ha notado sangre en su excremento? (ah naw-<u>tah</u>-daw <u>sahn</u>-greh ehn soo ehgs-kreh-<u>mehn</u>-taw)
Have you noticed blood in your urine?	¿Ha notado sangre en su orina? (ah naw-<u>tah</u>-daw <u>sahn</u>-greh ehn soo aw-r<u>ee</u>-nah)
Do you have pains in your stomach? When?	¿Sufre dolores de estómago? ¿Cuándo? (<u>soo</u>-freh daw-<u>law</u>-rehs deh ehs-<u>taw</u>-<u>mah</u>-gaw. <u>kwahn</u>-daw)
Do you take alcoholic beverages?	¿Toma usted bebidas alcohólicas? (<u>taw</u>-mah oos-tehd beh-<u>bee</u>-dahs ah<u>l</u>-kaw-<u>aw</u>-l<u>ee</u>-kahs)
- occasionally?	¿de vez en cuándo? (deh behs ehn <u>kwahn</u>-daw)
- frequently?	¿frecuentemente? (freh-kwehn-teh-<u>mehn</u>-teh)
- to excess?	¿excesivamente? (ehgs-seh-s<u>ee</u>-bah-<u>mehn</u>-teh)
Do you drink coffee, tea? How much?	¿Bebe café, té? ¿Cuánto? (<u>beh</u>-beh kah-<u>feh</u>, teh. <u>kwahn</u>-taw)
Do you smoke? How much?	¿Fuma usted? ¿Cuánto? (<u>foo</u>-mah oos-<u>tehd</u>. <u>kwahn</u>-taw)
Do you take any medicines, sedatives, tranquilizers?	¿Toma usted algunas medicinas, o algunos sedativos o calmantes? (<u>taw</u>-mah oos-tehd ahl-<u>goo</u>-nahs meh-d<u>ee</u>-s<u>ee</u>-nahs, aw ahl-<u>goo</u>-naws seh-<u>dah</u>-t<u>ee</u>-baws aw kahl-<u>mahn</u>-tehs)
What did your father die from?	¿De qué murió su padre? (deh keh moo-<u>ryaw</u> soo <u>pah</u>-dreh)
What did your mother die from?	¿De qué murió su madre? (deh keh moo-<u>ryaw</u> soo <u>mah</u>-dreh)
What chronic diseases have there been in your family?	¿Qué enfermedades crónicas han existido en su familia? (keh ehn-fehr-meh-<u>dah</u>-dehs <u>kraw</u>-n<u>ee</u>-kahs ahn ehg-s<u>ee</u>-st<u>ee</u>-daw ehn soo fah-m<u>ee</u>l-yah)
- epilepsy?	¿epilepsia? (eh-p<u>ee</u>-<u>lehp</u>-syah)
- diabetes?	¿diabetes? (d<u>ee</u>-ah-<u>beh</u>-tehs)
- heart?	¿corazón? (kaw-rah-<u>sawn</u>)
- high blood pressure?	¿presión alta de sangre? (preh-<u>syawn</u> <u>ahl</u>-tah deh <u>sahn</u>-greh)

- bronchitis?	¿bronquitis? (brawn-kēē-tēēs)
- tuberculosis?	¿tuberculosis? (too-behr-koo-law-sēēs)
- ulcers?	¿úlceras? (ool-seh-rahs)
Do you tire easily?	¿Se cansa fácilmente? (seh kahn-sah fah-sēēl-mehn-teh)
Do you have frequent headaches?	¿Sufre de dolor de cabeza frecuente-mente? (soo-freh deh daw-lawr deh kah-beh-sah freh-kwehn-teh-mehn-teh)
Do you ever feel numbness in any part of the body?	¿Siente alguna vez adormecimiento en alguna parte del cuerpo? (syehn-teh ahl-goo-nah behs ah-dawr-meh-sēē-myehn-taw ehn ahl-goo-nah pahr-teh dehl kwehr-paw)
Have you ever had any paralysis?	¿Ha tenido jamás alguna parálisis? (ah teh-nēē-daw hah-mahs ahl-goo-nah pah-rah-lēē-sēēs)
Have your eyes been examined recently?	¿Han sido examinados sus ojos recientemente? (ahn sēē-daw ehg-sah-mēē-nah-daws soos aw-haws reh-syehn-teh-mehn-teh)
Do you have blurring of vision?	¿Tiene ofuscación de la vista? (tyeh-neh aw-foos-kah-syawn deh lah bēē-stah)
Do you have double vision at times?	¿Tiene doble visión a veces? (tyeh-neh daw-bleh bēē-syawn ah beh-sehs)
Do you see spots in front of your eyes at times?	¿Ve usted puntos en frente de los ojos a veces? (beh oos-tehd poon-taws ehn frehn-teh deh laws aw-haws ah beh-sehs)
Do you use eyeglasses constantly?	¿Usa usted lentes (anteojos) con-stantemente? (oo-sah oos-tehd lehn-tehs [ahn-teh-aw-haws] kawn-stahn-teh-mehn-teh)
Do you hear well?	¿Oye bien? (aw-yeh byehn)
Do you hear buzzing noises in your ears at times?	¿Siente zumbidos en los oídos a veces? (syehn-teh soom-bēē-daws ehn laws aw-yēē-daws ah beh-sehs)
Do you have discharge from the ears at times?	¿Tiene secreciones en las orejas a veces? (tyeh-neh seh-kreh-syaw-nehs ehn lahs aw-reh-hahs ah beh-sehs)

Do you sometimes lose your balance?	¿A veces pierde usted el equilibrio? (ah beh-sehs pyehr-deh oos-tehd ehl eh-kee-lee-bryaw)
Do you have any unusual discharges from any part of your body?	¿Tiene usted algunas secreciones anormales en alguna parte del cuerpo? (tyeh-neh oos-tehd ahl-goo-nahs seh-kreh-syaw-nehs ah-nawr-mah-lehs ehn ahl-goo-nah pahr-teh dehl kwehr-paw)
Do you have a good appetite?	¿Tiene usted un buen apetito? (tyeh-neh oos-tehd oon bwehn ah-peh-tee-taw)
Do you feel any discomfort after eating?	¿Siente usted algún malestar del estómago después de comer? (syehn-teh oos-tehd ahl-goon mahl-ehs-tahr dehl ehs-taw-mah-gaw dehs-pwehs deh kaw-mehr)
- indigestion?	¿indigestión? (een-dee-hehs-tyawn)
- flatulence? (gas)	¿flatulencia? (flah-too-lehn-syah [gahs])
- pain?	¿dolor? (daw-lawr)
- often?	¿frecuentemente? (freh-kwehn-teh-mehn-teh)
Do you have allergies? To what? Foods? Medicines? Other?	¿Tiene alergias? ¿A qué? ¿Ciertos comestibles? ¿Medicinas?¿Otras? (tyeh-neh ah-lehr-hyahs. ah keh. syehr-taws kaw-mehs-tee-blehs. meh-dee-see-nahs. aw-trahs)
Have you ever had any venereal diseases? Syphilis? Gonorrhea? When?	¿Ha tenido jamás alguna enfermedad venérea? Sífilis? Gonorrea? Cuándo? (ah teh-nee-daw hah-mahs ahl-goo-nah ehn-fehr-meh-dahd beh-neh-ryah. see-fee-lees. gaw-naw-reh-yah. kwahn-daw)
Does it hurt when I press here?	¿Le duele cuando le aprieto aquí? (leh dweh-leh kwahn-daw leh ah-pryeh-taw ah-kee)
Have you ever had an operation?	¿Ha jamás sido operado (operada)? (ah hah-mahs see-daw aw-peh-rah-daw [aw-peh-rah-dah])
For what? When?	¿Para qué? ¿Cuándo? (pah-rah keh. kwahn-daw)
Have you ever had pernicious anaemia?	¿Ha tenido jamás anemia perniciosa? (ah teh-nee-daw hah-mahs ah-neh-myah pehr-nee-syaw-sah)
What illnesses have there been in your family?	¿Que enfermedades ha tenido su familia? (keh ehn-fehr-meh-dah-dehs ah teh-nee-daw soo fah-meel-yah)

GENERAL MEDICAL INTERVIEW	ENTREVISTA MÉDICA GENERAL (ehn-treh-bees-tah meh-dee-kah heh-neh-rahl)
Useful Vocabulary	Vocabulario Útil (baw-kah-boo-lah-ryaw oo-teel)
abdominal surgery	cirugía abdominal (see-roo-hee-ah ahb-daw-mee-nahl)
abnormal	anormal (ah-nawr-mahl)
allergy	la alergia (lah ah-lehr-hyah)
anaemia (pernicious)	la anemia (perniciosa) (lah ah-neh-myah [pehr-nee-syaw-sah])
appendicitis	la apendicitis (lah ah-pehn-dee-see-tees)
appetite	el apetito (ehl ah-peh-tee-taw)
balance	el equilibrio (ehl eh-kee-lee-bryaw)
barium test	la prueba de bario (lah prweh-bah deh bah-ryaw)
(to) bleed	sangrar (sahn-grahr)
blood	sangre (sahn-greh)
blood pressure	la presión de sangre (lah preh-syawn deh sahn-greh)
- high	alta (ahl-tah)
- low	baja (bah-hah)
body	el cuerpo (ehl kwehr-paw)
bronchitis	la bronquitis (lah brawn-kee-tees)
cancer	el cáncer (ehl kahn-sehr)
cardiogram	el cardiograma (ehl kahr-dyaw-grah-mah)
chronic disease	la enfermedad crónica (lah ehn-fehr-meh-dahd kraw-nee-kah)
clinic	la clínica (lah klee-nee-kah)
constipation	el estreñimiento (ehl ehs-treh-nyee-myehn-taw)
(to) consult	consultar (kawn-sool-tahr)
death	la muerte (lah mwehr-teh)
diabetes	la diabetes (lah dyah-beh-tehs)
diarrhea	la diarrea (lah dyah-reh-ah)

(to) die	morir (maw-<u>reer</u>)
discharge	la secreción; el derrame (lah seh-kreh-<u>syawn</u>; ehl deh-<u>rah</u>-meh)
dizziness	el vértigo (ehl behr-<u>tee</u>-gaw)
doctor's office...	el consultorio (ehl kawn-sool-<u>taw</u>-ryaw)
(to) eat	comer (kaw-<u>mehr</u>)
(to) eliminate	eliminar (eh-<u>lee</u>-mee-<u>nahr</u>)
epilepsy	la epilepsia (lah eh-p<u>ee</u>-<u>lehp</u>-syah)
(to) examine	examinar (ehg-sah-m<u>ee</u>-<u>nahr</u>)
exercise	el ejercicio (ehl eh-hehr-s<u>ee</u>-syaw)
external use	uso externo (<u>oo</u>-saw ehgs-<u>tehr</u>-naw)
eyes	los ojos (laws <u>aw</u>-haws)
eyeglasses	las gafas; las lentes; los anteojos (lahs <u>gah</u>-fahs; lahs <u>lehn</u>-tehs; laws ahn-teh-<u>aw</u>-haws)
fat	grueso (masculine) (<u>grweh</u>-saw) gruesa (feminine) (<u>grweh</u>-sah)
flatulence	el gas (ehl gahs)
food	el alimento (ehl ah-l<u>ee</u>-<u>mehn</u>-taw)
frequently	a menudo (ah meh-<u>noo</u>-daw)
(to) gain	ganar (gah-<u>nahr</u>)
gall stone	cálculo biliar (<u>kahl</u>-koo-law b<u>ee</u>-<u>lyahr</u>)
gastric ulcer	úlcera gástrica (<u>ool</u>-seh-rah <u>gahs</u>-tr<u>ee</u>-kah)
gauze	la gasa (lah <u>gah</u>-sah)
general rundown feeling	la lasitud (lah lah-s<u>ee</u>-<u>tood</u>)
headache	el dolor de cabeza (ehl daw-<u>lawr</u> deh kah-<u>beh</u>-sah)
hearing	el sentido del oído (ehl sehn-t<u>ee</u>-daw dehl aw-<u>ee</u>-daw)
heart	el corazón (ehl kaw-rah-<u>sawn</u>)
heartburn	la acedía (lah ah-seh-d<u>ee</u>-ah)
hernia	la hernia (lah <u>ehr</u>-nyah)

immunity	la inmunidad (lah ēēn-moo-nēē-dahd)
indigestion	la indigestión (lah ēēn-dēē-hehs-tyawn)
infectious	infeccioso (ēēn-fehk-syaw-saw)
insomnia	la insomnia (lah ēēn-sawm-nyah)
laboratory	el laboratorio (ehl lah-baw-rah-taw-ryaw)
(to) lose weight	perder peso (pehr-dehr peh-saw)
lungs	los pulmones (laws pool-maw-nehs)
malnutrition	la desnutrición (lah dehs-noo-trēē-syawn)
mumps	la papera (lah pah-peh-rah)
nausea	la náusea (lah nah-oo-seh-ah)
nervous	nervioso (masculine) (nehr-byaw-saw) nerviosa (feminine) (nehr-byaw-sah)
nervousness	la nerviosidad (lah nehr-byaw-sēē-dahd)
numbness	el adormecimiento (ehl ah-dawr-meh-sēē-myehn-taw)
obesity	el sobrepeso (ehl saw-breh-peh-saw)
operation	la operación (lah aw-peh-rah-syawn)
painful	doloroso (daw-law-raw-saw)
perspiration	la perspiración (lah pehr-spēē-rah-syawn)
prostate gland	la glándula de la próstata (lah glahn-doo-lah deh lah praw-stah-tah)
pulse	el pulso (ehl pool-saw)
relapse	la recaída (lah reh-kah-ēē-dah)
rheumatism	el reumatismo (ehl reh-oo-mah-tēēz-maw)
slipped disc	el disco desplazado (ehl dēēs-kaw dehs-plah-sah-daw)
sprain	la torcedura (lah tawr-seh-doo-rah)
stethoscope	el estetoscopio (ehl ehs-teh-taw-skaw-pyaw)

stomach	el estómago (ehl ehs-<u>taw</u>-mah-gaw)
stools	los heces; el excremento (laws eh-sehs; ehl ehgs-kreh-<u>mehn</u>-taw)
surgery	la cirugía (lah s<u>ee</u>-roo-<u>hee</u>-ah)
swollen	hinchado (<u>ee</u>n-<u>chah</u>-daw)
symptoms	los síntomas (laws s<u>ee</u>n-taw-mahs)
syphilis	la sífilis (lah s<u>ee</u>-f<u>ee</u>-l<u>ee</u>s)
thermometer	el termómetro (ehl tehr-<u>maw</u>-meh-traw)
thin	delgado; flaco (masculine) (dehl-<u>gah</u>-daw; <u>flah</u>-kaw) delgada; flaca (feminine) (dehl-<u>gah</u>-dah; <u>flah</u>-kah)
(to) tire	cansarse (kahn-<u>sahr</u>-seh)
(to be) tired	estar cansado (masculine) (kahn-<u>sah</u>-daw) estar cansada (feminine) (kahn-<u>sah</u>-dah)
tremor	el temblor (ehl tehm-<u>blawr</u>)
tumor	el tumor (ehl too-<u>mawr</u>)
(to) urinate	orinar (aw-r<u>ee</u>-<u>nahr</u>)
vaccine	la vacuna (lah bah-<u>koo</u>-nah)
venereal disease	la enfermedad venérea (lah ehn-fehr-meh-<u>dahd</u> beh-neh-ryah)
vision	la vista (lah b<u>ee</u>s-tah)
weak	débil (<u>deh</u>-b<u>ee</u>l)
weight	el peso (ehl <u>peh</u>-saw)
X-rays	los rayos equis (laws <u>rah</u>-yaws eh-k<u>ee</u>s)

BBB

X-RAYS

X-RAYS	RAYOS EQUIS (rah-yaws eh-kees)
Stay calm!	¡Quédese calmo (calma)! (keh-deh-seh kahl-maw [kahl-mah])
Please undress and put on this gown.	Favor de quitarse la ropa y de ponerse esta bata. (fah-bawr deh kee-tahr-seh lah raw-pah ee deh paw-nehr-seh ehs-tah bah-tah)
Please wait here (there) until we call you.	Por favor, espere usted aquí (allí) hasta que lo (la) llamemos. (pawr fah-bawr ehs-peh-reh oos-tehd ah-kee [ah-yee] ahs-tah keh law [lah] yah-meh-maws)
We shall be with you shortly.	Lo (la) atenderemos dentro de unos minutos. (law [lah] ah-tehn-deh-reh-maws dehn-traw deh oo-naws mee-noo-taws)
Sit on this table with your legs hanging over the side.	Siéntese en esta mesa con las piernas pendientes al lado de la mesa. (syehn-teh-seh ehn ehs-tah meh-sah kawn lahs pyehr-nahs pehn-dyehn-tehs ahl lah-daw deh lah meh-sah)
Remain perfectly still.	Quédese perfectamente inmóvil. (keh-deh-seh pehr-fehk-tah-mehn-teh een-maw-beel)
Please drink this liquid slowly.	Favor de beber este líquido despacio. (fah-bawr deh beh-behr ehs-teh lee-kee-daw dehs-pah-syaw)
Take a deep breath and hold it.	Respire hondo y mantenga la respiración. (rehs-pee-reh awn-daw ee mahn-tehn-gah lah rehs-pee-rah-syawn)
Breathe out.	Exhale. (ehg-sah-leh)
Now breathe normally.	Ahora respire normalmente. (ah-aw-rah rehs-pee-reh nawr-mahl-mehn-teh)
Repeat, please.	Repita, por favor. (reh-pee-tah pawr fah-bawr)
Please lie down on the table.	Por favor, acuéstese en la mesa. (pawr fah-bawr, ah-kwehs-teh-seh ehn lah meh-sah)
- on your stomach	boca abajo (baw-kah ah-bah-haw)
- on you back	boca arriba (baw-kah ah-ree-bah)

- on your left side	sobre el lado izquierdo (saw-breh ehl lah-daw ees-kyehr-daw)
- on your right side	sobre el lado derecho (saw-breh ehl lah-daw deh-reh-chaw)
Don't move!	¡No se mueva! (naw seh mweh-bah)
Please maintain each position in which we place you.	Por favor, mantenga cada posición en que lo (la) pongamos. (pawr fah-bawr mahn-tehn-gah kah-dah paw-see-syawn ehn keh law[lah] pawn-gah-maws)
Bend your left (right) arm.	Doble el brazo izquierdo (derecho). (daw-bleh ehl brah-saw ees-kyehr-daw [deh-reh-chaw])
- your left (right) knee	la rodilla izquierda (derecha) (lah raw-dee-yah ees-kyehr-dah [deh-reh-chah])
- your head to the left	la cabeza a la izquierda (lah kah-beh-sah ah lah ees-kyehr-dah)
- to the right	a la derecha (ah lah deh-reh-chah)
- forward	sobre el pecho (saw-breh ehl peh-chaw)
- backward	por atrás (pawr ah-trahs)
Lift your head!	¡Levante la cabeza! (leh-bahn-teh lah kah-beh-sah)
- your right arm	el brazo derecho (ehl brah-saw deh-reh-chaw)
- your left arm	el brazo izquierdo (ehl brah-saw ees-kyehr-daw)
- your right leg	la pierna derecha (lah pyehr-nah deh-reh-chah)
- your left leg	la pierna izquierda (lah pyehr-nah ees-kyehr-dah)
- both legs	las dos piernas (lahs daws pyehr-nahs)
- both arms	los dos brazos (laws daws brah-saws)
Stand up!	¡Levántese! (leh-bahn-teh-seh)
Face the machine!	¡Encárese al aparato! (ehn-kah-reh-seh ahl ah-pah-rah-taw)

Remain perfectly still!

¡Quédese perfectamente inmóvil! (keh-deh-seh pehr-fehk-tah-mehn-teh een-maw-beel)

Turn to the left!

¡Vuélvase a la izquierda! (bwehl-bah-seh ah lah ees-kyehr-dah)

Turn your back to the machine.

Vuelva la espalda al aparato. (bwehl-bah lah ehs-pahl-dah ahl ah-pah-rah-taw)

Stop! Hold that position!

¡Deténgase! ¡Mantenga esa posición! (deh-tehn-gah-seh. mahn-tehn-gah eh-sah paw-see-syawn)

The X-rays are finished.

Los rayos equis son terminados. (laws rah-yaws eh-kees sawn tehr-mee-nah-daws)

Thank you for your cooperation.

Gracias por su cooperación. (grah-syahs pawr soo kaw-aw-pehr-ah-syawn)

You may now get down from the table.

Ahora puede bajarse de la mesa. (ah-aw-rah pweh-deh bah-hahr-seh deh lah meh-sah)

Move on to the stretcher!

¡Muévase sobre la camilla! (mweh-bah-seh saw-breh lah kah-mee-yah)

Be careful!

¡Cuidado! (kwee-dah-daw)

Return to your wheelchair.

Regrese a la silla de ruedas. (reh-greh-seh ah lah see-yah deh rweh-dahs)

They will take you to your room shortly.

Lo (la) van a llevar a su cuarto dentro de unos minutos. (law [lah] bahn ah yeh-bahr ah soo kwahr-taw dehn-traw deh oo-naws mee-noo-taws)

X-RAYS

LOS RAYOS EQUIS (laws rah-yaws eh-kees)

Useful Vocabulary

Vocabulario Útil (baw-kah-boo-lah-ryaw oo-teel)

(to) assist

ayudar (ah-yoo-dahr)

(to) attend

atender (ah-tehn-dehr)

back

la espalda (lah ehs-pahl-dah)

(to) bend

doblar (daw-blahr)

(to) breathe

respirar (rehs-pee-rahr)

(to) call

llamar (yah-mahr)

Calm yourself!

¡Cálmese! (kahl-meh-seh)

Be careful!	¡Cuidado! (kwēē-<u>dah</u>-daw)
department	el departamento (ehl deh-pahr-tah-<u>mehn</u>-taw)
(to) drink	beber (beh-<u>behr</u>)
(to) exhale	exhalar (ehg-sah-<u>lahr</u>)
(to) finish	terminar; acabar (tehr-mēē-<u>nahr</u>. ah-kah-<u>bahr</u>)
(to) get down	bajar (bah-<u>hahr</u>)
(to) go up	subir (soo-<u>bēēr</u>)
head	la cabeza (lah kah-<u>beh</u>-sah)
inhale	inhalar (<u>ēēn</u>-ah-<u>lahr</u>)
(to) lift	levantar (leh-bahn-<u>tahr</u>)
liquid	el líquido (ehl <u>lēē</u>-<u>kēē</u>-daw)
machine	el aparato (ehl ah-pah-<u>rah</u>-taw)
maintain	mantener (mahn-teh-<u>nehr</u>)
pictures	las pinturas (lahs <u>pēēn</u>-<u>too</u>-rahs)
(to) put on	ponerse (paw-<u>nehr</u>-seh)
(to) sit down	sentarse (sehn-<u>tahr</u>-seh)
slowly	despacio (dehs-<u>pah</u>-syaw)
(to) stand up	levantarse (leh-bahn-<u>tahr</u>-seh)
stomach	el estómago (ehl ehs-<u>taw</u>-mah-gaw)
stretcher	la camilla (lah kah-<u>mēē</u>-yah)
table	la mesa (lah <u>meh</u>-sah)
(to) take off	quitarse (kee-<u>tahr</u>-seh)
technician	el técnico (ehl <u>tek</u>-<u>nēē</u>-kaw)
tests	las investigaciones (lahs <u>ēēn</u>-behs-<u>tēē</u>-gah-<u>syaw</u>-nehs)
(to) wait	esperar (ehs-peh-<u>rahr</u>)
wheelchair	la silla de ruedas (lah <u>see</u>-yah deh <u>rweh</u>-dahs)
X-rays	los rayos equis (laws <u>rah</u>-yaws eh-<u>kēēs</u>)

FINANCIAL ASSISTANCE

FINANCIAL ASSISTANCE	AYUDA FINANCIERA (ah-yoo-dah fee-nahn-syeh-rah)
What is your name?	¿Cuál es su nombre? (kwahl ehs soo nawm-breh)
What is your address?	¿Cuál es su dirección? (kwahl ehs soo dee-rehk-syawn)
What is your telephone number?	¿Cuál es su número de teléfono? (kwahl ehs soo noo-meh-raw deh teh-leh-faw-naw)
Do you live in a private home or an apartment?	¿Vive usted en una casa particular o en un apartamento? (bee-beh oos-tehd ehn oo-nah kah-sah pahr-tee-koo-lahr aw ehn oon ah-pahr-tah-mehn-taw)
Where were you born?	¿Dónde nació usted? (dawn-deh nah-syaw oos-tehd)
Are you a U. S. citizen?	¿Es usted ciudadano de los Estados Unidos? (ehs oos-tehd syoo-dah-dah-naw deh laws ehs-tah-daws oo-nee-daws)
How long have you lived in the U. S.?	¿Cuánto tiempo hace que vive en los Estados Unidos? (kwahn-taw tyehm-paw ah-seh keh bee-beh ehn laws ehs-tah-daws oo-nee-daws)
Are you married?	¿Es usted casado (casada)? (ehs oos-tehd kah-sah-daw [kah-sah-dah])
Single?	¿Soltero? (masculine) (sawl-teh-raw) ¿Soltera? (feminine) (sawl-teh-rah)
Separated?	¿Separado? (masculine) (seh-pah-rah-daw) ¿Separada? (feminine) (seh-pah-rah-dah)
Divorced?	¿Divorciado? (masculine) (dee-bawr-syah-daw) ¿Divorciada? (feminine) (dee-bawr-syah-dah)
How many children do you have?	¿Cuántos hijos tiene usted? (kwahn-taws ee-haws tyeh-neh oos-tehd)
How many people do you support altogether?	¿Cuántas personas mantiene usted en todo? (kwahn-tahs pehr-saw-nahs mahn-tyeh-neh oos-tehd ehn taw-daw)

How much rent do you pay?	¿Cuánta renta paga usted? (kwahn-tah rehn-tah pah-gah oos-tehd)
Do you have any debts? How much?	¿Tiene usted deudas? ¿Cuántas? (tyeh-neh oos-tehd deh-oo-dahs. kwahn-tahs)
Do you own your home?	¿Es usted propietario de su casa? (ehs oos-tehd praw-pyeh-tah-ryaw deh soo kah-sah)
How much is the mortgage?	¿Cuánto es la hipoteca? (kwahn-taw ehs lah ee-paw-teh-kah)
Are you employed?	¿Está usted empleado? (ehs-tah oos-tehd ehm-pleh-ah-daw)
How much do you earn weekly?	¿Cuánto gana usted por semana? (kwahn-taw gah-nah oos-tehd pawr seh-mah-nah)
Do you have any other income?	¿Tiene usted algún otro ingreso? (tyeh-neh oos-tehd ahl-goon aw-traw een-greh-saw)
Do you have a savings account?	¿Tiene usted una cuenta de ahorros? (tyeh-neh oos-tehd oo-nah kwehn-tah deh ah-aw-raws)
In which bank? How much?	¿En qué banco? ¿Cuánto? (ehn keh bahn-kaw. kwahn-taw)
Do you receive welfare assistance?	¿Recibe usted ayuda del departamento de ayuda social? (reh-see-beh oos-tehd ah-yoo-dah dehl deh-pahr-tah-mehn-taw deh ah-yoo-dah saw-syahl)
Do you receive money from the government? Insurance? Compensation? Stocks? Other?	¿Recibe usted dinero del gobierno, de seguros, de la compensación, de acciones? ¿De otros? (reh-see-beh oos-tehd dee-neh-raw dehl gaw-byehr-naw, deh seh-goo-raws, deh lah kawm-pehn-sah-syawn, deh ahk-syaw-nehs. deh aw-traws)
Do you receive help from any friend or member of the family?	¿Recibe usted ayuda de algún amigo o de algún miembro de la familia? (reh-see-beh oos-tehd ah-yoo-dah deh ahl-goon ah-mee-gaw aw deh ahl-goon myehm-braw deh lah fah-meel-yah)
Sign here, please!	¡Firme aquí, por favor! (feer-meh ah-kee pawr fah-bawr)

FINANCIAL ASSISTANCE	AYUDA FINANCIERA (ah-yoo-dah fee-nahn-syeh-rah)
Useful Vocabulary	Vocabulario Útil (baw-kah-boo-lah-ryaw oo-teel)
address	la dirección (lah dee-rehk-syawn) el domicilio (ehl daw-mee-see-lyaw)
apartment	el apartamento (ehl ah-pahr-tah-mehn-taw)
bank	el banco (ehl bahn-kaw)
(to be) born	nacer (nah-sehr)
car	el coche (ehl kaw-cheh) el auto (ehl ah-oo-taw)
child	el niño (ehl nee-nyaw) el hijo (ehl ee-haw)
children	los niños (laws nee-nyaws) los hijos (laws ee-haws)
citizen	el ciudadano (masculine) (ehl syoo-dah-dah-naw) la ciudadana (feminine) (lah syoo-dah-dah-nah)
compensation	la compensación (lah kawm-pehn-sah-syawn)
daughter	la hija (lah ee-hah)
(to) earn	ganar (gah-nahr)
family	la familia (lah fah-meel-yah)
father	el padre (ehl pah-dreh)
friend	el amigo (masculine) (ehl ah-mee-gaw) la amiga (feminine) (lah ah-mee-gah)
grandfather	el abuelo (ehl ah-bweh-law)
grandmother	la abuela (lah ah-bweh-lah)
(to) have	tener (teh-nehr)
home relief	la ayuda del departamento de ayuda social (lah ah-yoo-dah dehl deh-pahr-tah-mehn-taw deh ah-yoo-dah saw-syahl)
insurance	el seguro (ehl seh-goo-raw)
(to) live	vivir (bee-beer)

loan	el préstamo (ehl prehs-tah-maw)
married	casado (masculine) (kah-sah-daw) casada (feminine) (kah-sah-dah)
mortgage	la hipoteca (lah ee-paw-teh-kah)
mother	la madre (lah mah-dreh)
name	el nombre (ehl nawm-breh)
number	el número (ehl noo-meh-raw)
(to) owe	deber (deh-behr)
(to) have debts	tener deudas (teh-nehr deh-oo-dahs)
owner	el dueño (ehl dwehn-yaw) el propietario (ehl praw-pyeh-tah-ryaw)
(to) pay	pagar (pah-gahr)
people	la gente (lah hehn-teh) las personas (lahs pehr-saw-nahs)
private house	la casa privada (lah kah-sah pree-bah-dah)
(to) receive	recibir (reh-see-beer)
rent	la renta (lah rehn-tah)
(to) rent	alquilar (ahl-kee-lahr)
salary	el sueldo (ehl swehl-daw)
savings account	la cuenta de ahorros (lah kwehn-tah deh ah-aw-raws)
(to) sign	firmar (feer-mahr)
son	el hijo (ehl ee-haw)
stocks	las acciones (lahs ahk-syaw-nehs)
(to) support	mantener (mahn-teh-nehr)
telephone	el teléfono (ehl teh-leh-faw-naw)
United States	los Estados Unidos (laws ehs-tah-daws oo-nee-daws)
weekly	por semana (pawr seh-mah-nah)

ALCOHOLISM

ALCOHOLISM	EL ALCOHOLISMO (ehl ahl-kaw-aw-lēēs-maw)
How old are you?	¿Cuántos años tiene? (kwahn-taws ahn-yaws tyeh-neh)
Are you married or single?	¿Es casado (casada) o soltero (soltera)? (ehs kah-sah-daw [kah-sah-dah] aw sawl-teh-raw [sawl-teh-rah])
Do you have children? How many?	¿Tiene hijos? ¿Cuántos? (tyeh-neh ēē-haws. kwahn-taws)
Do you live with your wife? Husband? Parents?	¿Vive con su mujer? ¿Su marido? ¿Sus padres? (bēē-beh kawn soo moo-hehr. soo mah-rēē-daw. soos pah-drehs)
Do your parents know that you drink excessively?	¿Saben sus padres que usted bebe excesivamente? (sah-behn soos pah-drehs keh oos-tehd beh-beh ehg-seh-sēē-bah-mehn-teh)
Are your parents alcoholic? Any other members of your family?	¿Son alcohólicos sus padres? ¿Algunos otros miembros de la familia? (sawn ahl-kaw-aw-lēē-kaws soos pah-drehs. ahl-goo-naws aw-traws myehm-braws deh lah fah-mēēl-yah)
Are you here of your own volition?	¿Está usted aquí de su propia voluntad? (ehs-tah oos-tehd ah-kēē deh soo praw-pyah baw-loon-tahd)
What sort of work do you do?	¿Qué clase de trabajo hace usted? (keh klah-seh deh trah-bah-haw ah-seh oos-tehd)
What is your employer's name?	¿Cuál es el nombre de su jefe? (kwahl ehs ehl nawm-breh deh soo heh-feh)
How long have you worked for him?	¿Desde hace cuándo trabaja con él? (dehz-deh ah-seh kwahn-daw trah-bah-hah kawn ehl)
Do you change jobs often?	¿Cambia empleo a menudo? (kahm-byah ehm-pleh-aw ah meh-noo-daw)
Do you get along well with your fellow workers?	¿Tiene buenas relaciones con sus compañeros de trabajo? (tyeh-neh bweh-nahs reh-lah-syaw-nehs kawn soos kawm-pah-nyeh-raws deh trah-bah-haw)

Do you have matrimonial (family) problems?	¿Tiene problemas matrimoniales (familiares)? (tyeh-neh praw-bleh-mahs mah-tree-maw-nyah-lehs [fah-meel-lyah-rehs])
Do you have other personal problems?	¿Tiene otros problemas personales? (tyeh-neh aw-traws praw-bleh-mahs pehr-saw-nah-lehs)
Are you a United States citizen?	¿Es usted ciudadano de los Estados Unidos? (ehs oos-tehd syoo-dah-dah-naw deh laws ehs-tah-daws oo-nee-daws)
What is your social security number?	¿Cuál es su número de seguro social? (kwahl ehs soo noo-meh raw deh seh-goo-raw saw-syahl)
Where were you born?	¿Dónde nació usted? (dawn-deh nah-syaw oos-tehd)
How long have you been in this country?	¿Desde hace cuándo que vive en este país? (dehz-dah ah-seh kwahn-daw keh bee-beh ehn ehs-teh pah-ees)
How long have you lived in New York?	¿Desde hace cuándo que vive en Nueva York? (dehz-deh ah-seh kwahn-daw keh bee-beh ehn nweh-bah yawrk)
Are you receiving welfare assistance?	¿Está recibiendo ayuda social? (ehs-tah reh-see-byehn-daw ah-yoo-dah saw-syahl)
Have you been treated for alcoholism before? By whom? How long?	¿Ha sido tratado para el alcoholismo antes? ¿Por quién? ¿Por cuánto tiempo? (ah see-daw trah-tah-daw pah-rah ehl ahl-kaw-aw-lees-maw ahn-tehs. pawr kyehn. pawr kwahn-taw tyehm-paw)
How much alcohol do you take per day?	¿Cuánto alcohol toma usted por día? (kwahn-taw al-kawl taw-mah oos-tehd pawr dee-ah)
How long have you been drinking this quantity?	¿Desde cuándo toma esta cantidad? (dehz-deh kwahn-daw taw-mah ehs-tah kahn-tee-dahd)
Have you suffered from delirium tremens?	¿Ha sufrido usted de delirium tremens (temblor de miembros)? (ah soo-free-daw oos-tehd deh deh-lee-ry-oom treh-mehnz [tehm-blawr deh myehm-braws])
Have you had numbness of arms or legs?	¿Ha tenido adormecimiento de los miembros? (ah teh-nee-daw ah-dawr-meh-see-myehn-taw deh laws myehm-braws)

The doctor will see you shortly.	El médico lo (la) atenderá dentro de unos minutos. (ehl meh-dee-kaw law [lah] ah-tehn-deh-rah dehn-traw deh oo-naws mee-noo-taws)
ALCOHOLISM	EL ALCOHOLISMO (ehl ahl-kaw-aw-lees-maw)
Useful Vocabulary	Vocabulario Útil (baw-kah-boo-lah-ryaw oo-teel)
alcohol	el alcohol (ehl ahl-kawl)
alcoholic drinks	las bebidas alcohólicas (lahs beh-bee-dahs ahl-kaw-aw-lee-kahs)
beer	la cerveza (lah sehr-beh-sah)
brandy	el aguardiente (ehl ah-gwahr-dyehn-teh)
cirrhosis of the liver	cirosis del hígado (see-raw-sees dehl ee-gah-daw)
delirium tremens	temblor de miembros (tehm-blawr deh myehm-braws)
depressed	deprimido (masculine) (deh-pree-mee-daw) deprimida (feminine) (deh-pree-mee-dah)
detoxification	detoxificación (deh-tawk-see-fee-kah-syawn)
(to) drink	beber (beh-behr); tomar (taw-mahr)
employer	el jefe (ehl heh-feh)
(to) fight	pelearse (peh-leh-ahr-seh)
intoxication	la borachera (lah baw-rah-cheh-rah)
job	el empleo; el trabajo (ehl ehm-pleh-aw. ehl trah-bah-haw)
liquor	el licor (ehl lee-kawr)
marital problems	problemas matrimoniales (praw-bleh-mahs mah-tree-maw-nyah-lehs)
married	casado (masculine) (kah-sah-daw) casada (feminine) (kah-sah-dah)
nervousness	la nerviosidad (lah nehr-byaw-see-dahd)
numbness	el adormecimiento (ehl ah-dawr-meh-see-myehn-taw)
parents	los padres (los pah-drehs)

personal problems	los problemas personales (laws praw-<u>bleh</u>-mahs pehr-saw-<u>nah</u>-lehs)
quantity of liquor	la cantidad de licor (lah kah-tee-<u>dahd</u> deh lee-<u>kawr</u>)
religious	religioso (masculine) (reh-lee-<u>hyaw</u>-saw)
	religiosa (feminine) (reh-lee-<u>hyaw</u>-sah)
responsibilities	las responsabilidades (lahs rehs-pawn-sah-bee-lee-<u>dah</u>-dehs)
single	soltero (masculine) (sawl-<u>teh</u>-raw)
	soltera (feminine) (sawl-<u>teh</u>-rah)
social security number	el número de seguro social (ehl <u>noo</u>-meh-raw deh seh-<u>goo</u>-raw saw-<u>syahl</u>)
stimulant	el estimulante (ehl ehs-tee-moo-<u>lahn</u>-teh)
unconscious	inconsciente (een-kawn-<u>syehn</u>-teh)
welfare aid	la ayuda social del gobierno (lah ah-<u>yoo</u>-dah saw-<u>syahl</u> dehl gaw-<u>byehr</u>-naw)
wine	el vino (ehl bee-naw)
(to) work	trabajar (trah-bah-<u>hahr</u>)

CCC

DRUG ADDICTION

DRUG ADDICTION	LA ADICCIÓN A LAS DROGAS (lah ah-dēēk-syawn ah lahs draw-gahs)
What is your name?	¿Cómo se llama usted? (kaw-maw seh yah-mah oos-tehd)
What is your address?	¿Cuál es su dirección? (kwahl ehs soo dēē-rehk-syawn)
What is your telephone number?	¿Cuál es su número de teléfono? (kwahl ehs soo noo-meh-raw deh teh-leh-faw-naw)
Where were you born?	¿Dónde nació? (dawn-deh nah-syaw)
Are you a citizen of the United States?	¿Es usted ciudadano (ciudadana) de los Estados Unidos? (ehs oos-tehd syoo-dah-dah-naw [syoo-dah-dah-nah] deh laws ehs-tah-daws oo-nēē-daws)
How long have you lived in this city?	¿Desde hace cuándo vive en esta ciudad? (dehz-deh ah-seh kwahn-daw bēē-beh ehn ehs-tah syoo-dahd)
How old are you?	¿Qué edad tiene? (keh eh-dahd tyeh-neh)
Are you here of your own volition?	¿Está usted aquí de su propia voluntad? (ehs-tah oos-tehd ah-kēē deh soo praw-pyah baw-loon-tahd)
When did you start taking drugs?	¿Cuándo empezó a tomar drogas? (kwahn-daw ehm-peh-saw ah taw-mahr draw-gahs)
What drugs are you taking regularly?	¿Qué drogas está tomando regular-mente? (keh draw-gahs ehs-tah taw-mahn-daw reh-goo-lahr-mehn-teh)
How much do you take per day?	¿Qué cantidad toma usted por día? (keh kahn-tēē-dahd taw-mah oos-tehd pawr dēē-ah)
How much does it cost you per day?	¿Cuánto le cuesta por día? (kwahn-taw leh kwehs-tah pawr dēē-ah)
Are you employed?	¿Está usted empleado? (ehs-tah oos-tehd ehm-pleh-ah-daw)
What kind of work do you do?	¿Qué clase de trabajo hace usted? (keh klah-seh deh trah-bah-haw ah-seh oos-tehd)

Who is your employer? Name of the company?	¿Quién es su jefe? ¿El nombre de la compañía? (kyehn ehs soo heh-feh. ehl nawm-breh deh lah kawm-pah-nyee-ah)
How long have you worked with him?	¿Cuánto tiempo hace que usted trabaja con él? (kwahn-taw tyehm-paw ah-seh keh oos-tehd trah-bah-hah kawn ehl)
How much do you earn per week?	¿Cuánto gana usted por semana? (kawhn-taw gah-nah oos-tehd pawr seh-mah-nah)
Are you married?	¿Está usted casado (casada)? (ehs-tah oos-tehd kah-sah-daw [kah-sah-dah])
Do you have children? How many?	¿Tiene hijos? ¿Cuántos? (tyeh-neh ee-haws. kwahn-taws)
Do you live with your family?	¿Vive con su familia? (bee-beh kawn soo fah-meel-yah)
Do you support your family?	¿Usted mantiene a su familia? (oos-tehd mahn-tyeh-neh ah soo fah-meel-yah)
Do you receive welfare assistance?	¿Recibe usted ayuda social? (reh-see-beh oos-tehd ah-yoo-dah saw-syahl)
Have you had treatment for drug addiction before?	¿Ha tenido tratamiento para la adicción a las drogas antes? (ah teh-nee-daw trah-tah-myehn-taw pah-rah lah ah-deek-syawn ah lahs draw-gahs ahn-tehs)
When? Where? For how long?	¿Cuándo? ¿Dónde? ¿Por cuánto tiempo? (kwahn-daw. dawn-deh. pawr kwahn-taw tyehm-paw)
Why did you start again?	¿Por qué empezó de nuevo? (pawr keh ehm-peh-saw deh nweh-baw)
Do you have many personal problems?	¿Tiene usted muchos problemas personales? (tyeh-neh oos-tehd moo-chaws praw-bleh-mahs pehr-saw-nah-lehs)
Do you have marital difficulties?	¿Tiene muchas dificultades matrimoniales? (tyeh-neh moo-chahs dee-fee-kool-tah dehs mah-tree-maw-nyah-lehs)
Have you ever been under the care of a psychiatrist?	¿Ha sido jamás bajo cuidado de un psiquiatra? (ah see-daw hah-mahs bah-haw kwee-dah-daw deh oon see-kyah-tra)

Why do you want to be cured of the addiction?	¿Por qué quiere curarse de la adicción? (pawr keh kyeh-reh koo-rahr-seh deh lah ah-deek-syawn)
How much does the habit cost you per day?	¿Cuánto le cuesta la adicción por día? (kwahn-taw leh kwehs-tah lah ah-deek-syawn pawr dee-ah)
Do you have any chronic diseases?	¿Tiene usted alguna enfermedad crónica? (tyeh-neh oos-tehd ahl-goo-nah ehn-fehr-meh-dahd kraw-nee-kah)
- diabetes?	diabetes? (dee-ah-beh-tehs)
- heart disease?	enfermedad de corazón? (ehn-fehr-meh-dahd deh kaw-rah-sawn)
- respiratory ailment?	enfermedad respiratoria? (ehn-fehr-meh-dahd rehs-pee-rah-taw-ryah)

DRUG ADDICTION	ADICCIÓN A LAS DROGAS (ah-deek-syawn ah lahs draw-gahs)
Useful Vocabulary	Vocabulario Útil (baw-kah-boo-lah-ryaw oo-teel)
acid	ácido (ah-see-daw)
addict	el adicto (ehl ah-deek-taw)
addiction	la adicción (lah ah-deek-syawn)
antitoxic	antitóxico (ahn-tee-tawk-see-kaw)
barbiturates	barbitúricos (bahr-bee-too-ree-kaws)
(to be) born	nacer (nah-sehr)
children	los niños; los hijos (laws neen-yaws; laws ee-haws)
chronic disease	la enfermedad crónica (lah ehn-fehr-meh-dahd kraw-nee-kah)
citizen of the United States	ciudadano de los Estados Unidos (syoo-dah-dah-naw deh laws ehs-tah-daws oo-nee-daws) ciudadana (feminine) (syoo-dah-dah-nah)
cocaine	la cocaína (lah kaw-kah-ee-nah)
(to) consult	consultar (kawn-sool-tahr)
(to) cost	costar (kaws-tahr)
(to) cure	curar (koo-rahr)

detoxification	la detoxificación (lah deh-tawk-see-fee-kah-syawn)
dose	la dosis, (lah daw-sees)
(to) earn (money)	ganar (dinero) (gah-nahr [dee-neh-raw])
(to be) employed	estar empleado (masculine) (ehs-tahr ehm-pleh-ah-daw) empleada (feminine) (ehm-pleh-ah-dah)
family	la familia (lah fah-meel-yah)
habit	la adicción (lah ah-deek-syawn)
heroin	la heroína (lah eh-raw-ee-nah)
hypodermic needle	la aguja hipodérmica (lah ah-goo-hah ee-paw-dehr-mee-kah)
marital problems	los problemas matrimoniales (laws praw-bleh-mahs mah-tree-maw-nyah-lehs)
marijuana	la mariguana (lah mah-ree-gwah-nah)
married	casado (masculine) (kah-sah-daw) casada (feminine) (kah-sah-dah)
morphine	la morfina (lah mawr-fee-nah)
narcotic	el narcótico (ehl nahr-kaw-tee-kaw)
opium	el opio (ehl aw-pyaw)
psychiatrist	el psiquiatra (ehl see-kyah-trah)
quantity	la cantidad (lah kahn-tee-dahd)
rehabilitation	la rehabilitación (lah reh-ah-bee-lee-tah-syawn)
remedy	el remedio (ehl reh-meh-dyaw)
salary	el salario; la paga; el sueldo (ehl sah-lah-ryaw; lah pah-gah; ehl swehl-daw)
stomach pains	dolores de estómago (daw-law-rehs deh ehs-taw-mah-gaw)
tranquilizer	el calmante (ehl kahl-mahn-teh)
veins	las venas (lahs beh-nahs)
welfare aid	la ayuda social (lah ah-yoo-dah saw-syahl)

ΦΦΦ

ABORTION

ABORTIONS	ABORTOS (ah-<u>bawr</u>-taws)
What is your name?	¿Cómo se llama usted? (kaw-maw seh <u>yah</u>-mah oos-<u>tehd</u>)
How old are you?	¿Cuántos años tiene usted? (<u>kwahn</u>-taws <u>ahn</u>-yaws <u>tyeh</u>-neh oos-<u>tehd</u>)
Are you married or single?	¿Está usted casada o soltera? (ehs-<u>tah</u> oos-<u>tehd</u> kah-<u>sah</u>-dah aw sawl-<u>teh</u>-rah)
With whom do you live?	¿Con quién vive usted? (kawn kyehn <u>bee</u>-beh oos-<u>tehd</u>)
What is your address?	¿Cuál es su dirección? (kwahl ehs soo <u>dee</u>-rehk-<u>syawn</u>)
What is your telephone number?	¿Cuál es su número de teléfono? (kwahl ehs soo <u>noo</u>-meh-raw deh teh-<u>leh</u>-faw-naw)
Are you employed? Where?	¿Está empleada? ¿Dónde? (ehs-<u>tah</u> ehm-pleh-<u>ah</u>-dah. <u>dawn</u>-deh)
Do you use any kind of contra- ceptives? The pill? The diaphragm? Others?	¿Usa contraceptivos de alguna clase? ¿La píldora? ¿El diafragma? ¿Otros? (oo-sah kawn-trah-sehp-<u>tee</u>-baws deh ahl-<u>goo</u>-nah klah-seh. lah <u>peel</u>-daw-rah. ehl <u>dee</u>-ah-frahg-mah. <u>aw</u>-traws)
How do you know you are pregnant?	¿Cómo lo sabe que está embarazada? (kaw-maw law <u>sah</u>-beh keh ehs-<u>tah</u> ehm-bah-rah-<u>sah</u>-dah)
Whom did you consult?	¿A quién consultó? (ah kyehn kawn-sool-<u>taw</u>)
When did your pregnancy start?	¿Cuándo empezó su embarazo? (kwahn-daw ehm-peh-<u>saw</u> <u>soo</u> ehm-bah-rah-saw)
How did you react when you found out you were pregnant?	¿Cómo reaccionó cuando supo que estaba embarazada? (<u>kaw</u>-maw reh-ahk-syaw-naw <u>kwahn</u>-daw <u>soo</u>-paw keh ehs-<u>tah</u>-bah ehm-bah-rah-<u>sah</u>-dah)
How did the baby's father react when you told him?	¿Cómo reaccionó el padre de la criatura cuando se lo dijo? (<u>kaw</u>-maw reh-ahk-syaw-<u>naw</u> ehl <u>pah</u>-dreh deh lah <u>kree</u>-ah-<u>too</u>-rah kwahn-daw seh law <u>dee</u>-haw)
How did your parents react when you told them?	¿Cómo reaccionaron sus padres cuando se lo dijo? (<u>kaw</u>-maw reh-ahk-syaw-nah-rawn soos <u>pah</u>-drehs <u>kwahn</u>-daw seh law <u>dee</u>-haw)

Do you want the baby?

¿Usted quiere tener la criatura?
(oos-tehd kyeh-reh teh-nehr lah
kree-ah-too-rah)

How are you going to support
the baby?

¿Cómo va a mantener al niño?
(kaw-maw bah ah mahn-teh-nehr
ahl neen-yaw)

Are you still having relations
with the father of your child?

¿Tiene relaciones todavía con el
padre de la criatura? (tyeh-neh
reh-lah-syaw-nehs taw-dah-bee-
ah kawn ehl pah-dreh deh lah cree-
ah-too-rah)

Does he want you to have an
abortion?

¿El quiere que usted tenga un aborto?
(ehl kyeh-reh keh oos-tehd tehn-
gah oon ah-bawr-taw)

Would he be willing to support the
baby if you do not have an
abortion?

¿Quisiera el padre mantener a la
criatura si usted no tuviera un aborto?
(kee-syeh-rah ehl pah-dreh mahn-
teh-nehr ah lah kree-ah-too-rah
see oos-tehd naw too-byeh-rah oon
ah-bawr-taw)

Would your parents help support
the baby if you do not have an
abortion?

¿Quisieran sus padres ayudar a
mantener a la criatura, si usted
no tuviera un aborto? (kee-syeh-
rahn soos pah-drehs ah-yoo-dahr
ah mahn-teh-nehr ah lah kree-ah-
too-rah see oos-tehd naw too-byeh-
rah oon ah-bawr-taw)

Do you have any other children?
How many?

¿Tiene otros niños? ¿Cuántos?
(tyeh-neh aw-traws neen-yaws.
kwahn-taws)

Do you receive welfare
assistance?

¿Recibe usted ayuda del gobierno?
(reh-see-beh oos-tehd ah-yoo-dah
dehl gaw-byehr-naw)

Have you had, or do you have,
any venereal disease?

¿Ha tenido, o tiene, alguna enfermedad
venérea? (ah teh-nee-daw, aw tyeh-
neh, ahl-goo-nah ehn-fehr-meh-
dahd beh-neh-ryah)

Do you take any drugs? Which?

¿Toma algunas drogas? ¿Cuáles?
(taw-mah ahl-goo-nahs draw-gahs.
kwah-lehs)

Do you definitely want this
abortion?

¿Quiere usted este aborto definitiva-
mente? (kyeh-reh oos-tehd ehs-
teh ah-bawr-taw deh-fee-nee-tee-
bah-mehn-teh)

Have you ever been treated for
any mental disorders?

¿Ha sido jamás tratada para algún
desorden mental? (hah see-daw
hah-mahs trah-tah-dah pah-rah
ahl-goon deh-sawr-dehn mehn-tahl)

Do you have any physical disabilities?	¿Tiene alguna incapacidad física? (tyeh-neh ahl-goo-nah een-kah-pah-see-dahd fee-see-kah)
Have you ever been under a doctor's care for any diseases?	¿Ha sido tratada por un médico para alguna enfermedad? (ah see-daw trah-tah-dah pawr oon meh-dee-kaw pah-rah ahl-goo-nah ehn-fehr-meh-dahd)
- diabetes?	¿diabetes? (dee-ah-beh-tehs)
- heart condition?	¿enfermedad del corazón? (ehn-fehr-meh-dahd dehl kaw-rah-sawn)
- rheumatic fever?	¿fiebre reumática? (fyeh-breh reh-oo-mah-tee-kah)
- other?	¿otra? (aw-trah)
Please bring in the following documents:	Favor de entregar los documentos siguientes. (fah-bawr deh ehn-treh-gahr laws daw-koo-mehn-taws see-ghyehn-tehs)
- birth certificate, or any other proof of age.	Certificado de nacimiento, o alguna otra comprobación de edad. (sehr-tee-fee-kah-daw deh nah-see-myehn-taw aw ahl-goo-nah aw-trah kawm-praw-bah-syawn deh eh-dahd)
- birth certificates of your other children.	Certificados de nacimiento de sus otros hijos. (sehr-tee-fee-kah-daws deh nah-see-myehn-taw deh soos aw-traws ee-haws)
- a statement from your landlord stating how much rent you pay.	Una declaración del dueño de la casa informándonos qué renta le paga usted. (oo-nah deh-klah-rah-syawn dehl dwehn-yaw deh lah kah-sah een-fawr-mahn-daw-naws keh rehn-tah leh pah-gah oos-tehd)
- a statement from your employer as to what salary he pays you.	Una declaración de su jefe sobre el sueldo que le paga. (oo-nah deh-klah-rah-syawn deh soo heh-feh saw-breh ehl swehl-daw keh leh pah-gah)
- a statement from your doctor as to why you cannot work.	Una declaración de su médico explicando la razón por la cual usted no puede trabajar. (oo-nah deh-klah-rah-syawn deh soo meh-dee-kaw eks-plee-kahn-daw lah rah-sawn pawr lah kwahl oos-tehd naw pweh-deh trah-bah-hahr)

ABORTION	EL ABORTO (ehl ah-<u>bawr</u>-taw)
Useful Vocabulary	Vocabulario Útil (baw-kah-boo-<u>lah</u>-ryaw <u>oo</u>-t<u>ee</u>l)
abortion	el aborto (ehl ah-<u>bawr</u>-taw)
address	la dirección (lah d<u>ee</u>-rehk-<u>syawn</u>)
anxiety	la ansia (lah <u>ahn</u>-syah)
apartment	el apartamento (ehl ah-pahr-tah- <u>mehn</u>-taw)
baby	el bebé; la criatura (ehl beh-beh; lah kr<u>ee</u>-ah-<u>too</u>-rah)
birth certificate	El certificado de nacimiento (ehl sehr-t<u>ee</u>-f<u>ee</u>-<u>kah</u>-daw deh nah-s<u>ee</u>- <u>myehn</u>-taw)
(to) care (for)	cuidar de (kw<u>ee</u>-<u>dahr</u> deh)
child	el hijo (masculine) (ehl <u>ee</u>-haw) la hija (feminine) (lah <u>ee</u>-hah)
children	los hijos (laws <u>ee</u>-haws)
condom	el condón (ehl kawn-<u>dawn</u>)
consult	consultar (kawn-sool-<u>tahr</u>)
contraceptive	el contraceptivo (ehl kawn-trah- sehp-t<u>ee</u>-baw)
delivery	el parto (ehl <u>pahr</u>-taw)
disease	la enfermedad (lah ehn-fehr-meh- <u>dahd</u>)
diaphragm	el diafragma (ehl d<u>ee</u>-ah-<u>frahg</u>-mah)
disability	la incapacidad (lah <u>een</u>-kah-pah-s<u>ee</u>- <u>dahd</u>)
document	el documento (ehl daw-koo-<u>mehn</u>- taw)
drugs	las drogas (lahs <u>draw</u>-gahs)
employer	el jefe (ehl <u>heh</u>-feh)
father	el padre (ehl <u>pah</u>-dreh)
foam (contraceptive)	la medicina espumosa (lah meh-d<u>ee</u>- <u>see</u>-nah ehs-poo-<u>maw</u>-sah)
husband	el esposo; el marido (ehl ehs-<u>paw</u>- saw; ehl mah-<u>ree</u>-daw)

illness	la enfermedad (lah ehn-fehr-meh-dahd)
job	el empleo (ehl ehm-pleh-yaw)
landlord	el dueño de la casa (ehl dwehn-yaw deh lah kah-sah)
(to) live	vivir (bee-beer)
lover	el amante (ehl ah-mahn-teh)
(to) marry	casarse con (kah-sahr-seh kawn)
married	estar casado (masculine) (ehs-tahr kah-sah-daw) estar casada (feminine) (ehs-tahr kah-sah-dah)
month	el mes (ehl mehs)
monthly	mensual (mehn-swahl)
parents	los padres (laws pah-drehs)
(to) own	ser propietario de (sehr praw-pyeh-tah-ryaw deh)
pregnancy	el embarazo (ehl ehm-bah-rah-saw)
pill	la píldora (lah peel-daw-rah)
rent	la renta (lah rehn-tah)
(to) rent	alquilar (ahl-kee-lahr)
sexual relations	relaciones sexuales (reh-lah-syaw-nehs sehk-swah-lehs)
single	soltera (feminine) (sawl-teh-rah) soltero (masculine) (sawl-teh-raw)
social service	la ayuda social (lah ah-yoo-dah saw-syahl)
social worker	consejero (a) de la ayuda social (kawn seh-heh-raw [rah] deh lah ah-yoo-dah saw-syahl)
(to) support	mantener (mahn-teh-nehr)
suppository	el supositorio (ehl soo-paw-see-taw-ryaw)
venereal disease	la enfermedad venérea (lah ehn-fehr-meh-dahd beh-neh-ryah)
(to) want	querer (keh-rehr)

welfare   la ayuda social (lah ah-<u>yoo</u>-dah saw-
                              syahl)

wife   la esposa; la mujer (lah ehs-<u>paw</u>-
                              sah.   lah moo-<u>hehr</u>)

work   el trabajo (ehl trah-<u>bah</u>-haw)

(to) work   trabajar (trah-bah-<u>hahr</u>)

ℬℬℬ

THE NURSE - GENERAL

THE NURSE	LA ENFERMERA (lah ehn-fehr-<u>meh</u>-rah)
Good morning!	¡Buenos días! (bweh-naws <u>dee</u>-ahs)
I will be your nurse for today.	Yo seré su enfermera para hoy. (yaw seh-<u>reh</u> soo ehn-fehr-<u>meh</u>- rah pah-<u>rah</u> awy)
How do you feel today?	¿Cómo se siente hoy? (<u>kaw</u>-maw seh <u>syehn</u>-teh awy)
Did you sleep well last night?	¿Durmió bien anoche? (door-<u>myaw</u> byehn ah-<u>naw</u>-cheh)
Do you have any pain? Where?	¿Tiene usted algún dolor? ¿Dónde? (<u>tyeh</u>-neh oos-<u>tehd</u> ahl-<u>goon</u> daw- <u>lawr</u>. dawn-<u>deh</u>)
Are you comfortable?	¿Está usted cómodo (cómoda)? (ehs-<u>tah</u> oos-tehd <u>kaw-maw-daw</u> [<u>kaw-maw-dah</u>])
Would you like me to open the window?	¿Quiere que le abra la ventana? (<u>kyeh</u>-reh keh leh <u>ah</u>-brah lah behn- <u>tah</u>-nah)
Do you need the bed pan?	¿Necesita la silleta? (neh-seh- <u>see</u>-tah lah <u>see</u>-yeh-tah)
Let me take your temperature.	Déjeme tomar su temperatura. (deh-heh-meh taw-<u>mahr</u> soo tehm) peh-rah-<u>too</u>-rah)
I am going to take your blood pressure.	Voy a tomarle la presión de sangre. (bawy ah taw-<u>mahr</u>-leh lah preh- syawn deh <u>sahn</u>-greh)
Make a fist.	¡Haga un puno! (<u>ah</u>-gah oon <u>poon</u>-yaw)
Have you voided?	¿Ha orinado usted? (ah aw-<u>ree</u>-nah- daw oos-<u>tehd</u>)
Have you had a bowel movement?	¿Ha eliminado? (ah eh-<u>lee</u>-<u>mee</u>-nah- daw)
Are you constipated?	¿Está usted estreñido (estreñida)? (ehs-tah oos-<u>tehd</u> ehs-trehn-<u>yee</u>- daw [ehs-trehn-<u>yee</u>-dah])
I shall have to give you an enema.	Tengo que darle una lavativa. (tehn- gaw keh <u>dahr</u>-leh <u>oo</u>-nah lah-<u>bah</u>- <u>tee</u>-bah)
Please take these pills.	Por favor, tome estas píldoras. (pawr fah-<u>bawr</u> <u>taw</u>-meh ehs-tahs <u>peel</u>-daw-rahs)

Please take this medicine.
Por favor, tome esta medicina.
(pawr fah-bawr taw-meh ehs-tah
meh-dee-see-nah)

Drink plenty of water.
Beba bastante agua. (beh-bah bahs-
tahn-teh ah-gwah)

I shall be back shortly to give
you a bath.
Regresaré dentro de poco para darle
un baño. (reh-greh-sah-reh dehn-
traw deh paw-kaw pah-rah dahr-leh
oon bahn-yaw)

Have a good breakfast.
Tome un buen desayuno. (taw-meh
oon bwehn deh-sah-yoo-naw)

THE BATH

EL BAÑO
(ehl bahn-yaw)

Lift your arm!
¡Levante el brazo! (leh-bahn-teh
ehl brah-saw)

Lift your leg!
¡Levante la pierna! (leh-bahn-teh
lah pyehr-nah)

Turn over on your right side!
¡Voltéese al lado derecho! (bawl-
teh-eh-seh ahl lah-daw deh-reh-
chaw)

Turn over on your left side!
¡Voltéese al lado izquierdo! (bawl-
teh-eh-seh ahl lah-daw ees-kyehr-
daw)

Lie on your back!
¡Acuéstese boca arriba! (ah-kwehs-
teh-seh baw-kah ah-ree-bah)

Lie on your stomach!
¡Acuéstese boca abajo! (ah-kwehs-
teh-seh baw-kah ah-bah-haw)

Would you like me to comb
your hair?
¿Quisiera que le peine el pelo?
(kee-syeh-rah keh leh peh-ee-neh
ehl peh-law)

Where is your comb?
¿Dónde está su peine? (dawn-deh
ehs-tah soo peh-ee-neh)

Would you like me to rub your
back with alcohol?
¿Quisiera que le frote la espalda
con alcohol? (kee-syeh-rah keh
leh fraw-teh lah ehs-pahl-dah kawn
ahl-kawl)

Would you like me to change
your nightgown (pajamas)?
¿Quisiera que le cambie el camisón
(el pijama)? (kee-syeh-rah keh leh
kahm-byeh ehl kah-mee-sawn [ehl
pee-hah-mah])

The doctor said you may get out of bed for a while today.	El médico ha dicho que usted puede levantarse hoy por un rato. (ehl meh-dee-kaw ah dee-chaw keh oos-tehd pweh-deh leh-bahn-tahr-seh awy pawr oon rah-taw)
I am going to change your bed linen.	Voy a cambiar las sábanas. (bawy ah kahm-byahr lahs sah-bah-nahs)
Would you like to sit in the chair?	¿Quisiera sentarse en la silla? (kee syeh-rah sehn-tahr-seh ehn lah see-yah)
Would you like another blanket?	¿Quisiera otra frasada? (kee-syeh-rah aw-trah frah-sah-dah)
Would you like to go to the bathroom?	¿Quisiera ir al cuarto de baño? (kee-syeh-rah eer ahl kwahr-taw deh bahn-yaw)
The doctor will visit you shortly.	El médico le (la) visitará dentro de poco. (ehl meh-dee-kaw le [lah] bee-see-tah-rah dehn-traw deh paw-kaw)
Shall I raise your bed?	¿Levanto su cabecera? (leh-bahn-taw soo kah-beh-seh-rah)
Do you have a robe and slippers?	¿Tiene una bata y pantuflas? (tyeh-neh oo-nah bah-tah ee pahn-too-flahs)
If you need anything, press the buzzer.	Si necesita algo, apriete el timbre. (see neh-seh-see-tah ahl-gaw ah-pryeh-teh ehl teem-breh)
THE NURSE	LA ENFERMERA (lah ehn-fehr-meh-rah)
Useful Vocabulary	Vocabulario Útil (baw-kah-boo-lah-ryaw oo-teel)
absorbent cotton	el algodón absorbente (ehl ahl-gaw-dawn ahb-sawr-behn-teh)
adhesive tape	el esparadrapo (ehl ehs-pah-rah-drah-paw)
aspirin	la aspirina (lah ahs-pee-ree-nah)
back	la espalda (lah ehs-pahl-dah)
bath	el baño (ehl bahn-yaw)
bed	la cama (lah kah-mah)
bed clothes	la ropa de cama (lah raw-pah deh kah-mah)
bedpan	la silleta (lah see-yeh-tah)

blanket	la manta; la frasada (lah mahn-tah; lah frah-sah-dah)
blood plasma	plasma sanguíneo (plahz-mah sahn-gee-neh-aw)
blood pressure	la presión de sangre (lah preh-syawn deh sahn-greh)
breakfast	el desayuno (ehl deh-sah-yoo-naw)
buzzer	el timbre (ehl teem-breh)
capsule	la cápsula (lah kahp-soo-lah)
(to) change	cambiar (kahm-byahr)
(to) close	cerrar (seh-rahr)
(to be) cold	tener frío (teh-nehr free-aw)
comb	el peine (ehl pehy-neh)
(to) comb	peinar (pehy-nahr)
comfortable	cómodo (masculine) (kaw-maw-daw) cómoda (feminine) (kaw-maw-dah)
convalescent	convaleciente (kawn-bah-leh-syehn-teh)
dinner	la cena (lah seh-nah)
doctor	el médico (ehl meh-dee-kaw)
(to) draw the curtains	descorrer las cortinas (dehs-kaw-rehr lahs kawr-tee-nahs)
dressing	la curación (lah koo-rah-syawn)
(to) drink	beber, tomar (beh-behr, taw-mahr)
(to) eat	comer (kaw-mehr)
enema	la enema; la lavativa (lah eh-neh-mah; lah lah-bah-tee-bah)
fist (to make a)	hacer un puño (ah-sehr oon poon-yaw)
glucose	la glucosa (lah gloo-kaw-sah)
gown	el camisón (ehl kah-mee-sawn)
hairbrush	el cepillo para el pelo (ehl seh-pee-yaw pah-rah ehl peh-law)
(to be) hot	tener calor (teh-nehr kah-lawr)

injection	la inyección (lah <u>ee</u>n-yehk-<u>syawn</u>)
intravenous	intravenoso (<u>ee</u>n-trah-beh-<u>naw</u>-saw)
laxative	el purgante (ehl poor-<u>gahn</u>-teh)
left side	el lado izquierdo (ehl <u>lah</u>-daw <u>ee</u>s-<u>kyehr</u>-daw)
(to) lift	levantar (leh-bahn-<u>tahr</u>)
light (to put out the)	apagar la luz (ah-pah-<u>gahr</u> lah loos)
lotion	la loción (lah law-<u>syawn</u>)
(to) lower the head of the bed	bajar la cabecera (bah-<u>hahr</u> lah kah-beh-<u>seh</u>-rah)
lunch	el almuerzo (ehl ahl-<u>mwehr</u>-saw)
(to) lunch	almorzar (ahl-mawr-<u>sahr</u>)
magnesia	la magnesia (lah mahg-<u>neh</u>-syah)
massage	el masaje (ehl mah-<u>sah</u>-heh)
mattress	el colchón (ehl kawl-<u>chawn</u>)
(to) open	abrir (ah-br<u>ee</u>r)
- the window	la ventana (lah behn-<u>tah</u>-nah)
- the door	la puerta (lah <u>pwehr</u>-tah)
oxygen	el oxígeno (ehl awk-s<u>ee</u>-heh-naw)
pain	el dolor (ehl daw-<u>lawr</u>)
pill	la píldora (lah p<u>eel</u>-daw-rah)
Press the buzzer!	¡ Apriete el timbre! (ah-<u>pryeh</u>-teh ehl t<u>ee</u>m-breh)
pajamas	el pijama (ehl p<u>ee</u>-hah-mah)
(to) raise the head of the bed	elevar la cabecera (eh-leh-<u>bahr</u> lah kah-beh-<u>seh</u>-rah)
right side	el lado derecho (ehl <u>lah</u>-daw deh-<u>reh</u>-chaw)
robe	la bata (lah <u>bah</u>-tah)
(to) rub	frotar (fraw-<u>tahr</u>)
sedative	el calmante (ehl kahl-<u>mahn</u>-teh) el sedativo (ehl seh-dah-<u>tee</u>-baw)
sheets	las sábanas (lahs <u>sah</u>-bah-nahs)

(to) sit up	incorporarse (ēēn-kawr-paw-<u>rahr</u>-seh)
(to) sit down	sentarse (sehn-<u>tahr</u>-seh)
(to) sleep	dormir (dawr-<u>mēēr</u>)
slippers	las pantuflas (lahs pahn-<u>too</u>-flahs)
(to) swallow	tragar (trah-<u>gahr</u>)
talcum powder	el polvo de talco (ehl <u>pawl</u>-baw deh <u>tahl</u>-kaw)
temperature	la temperatura (lah tehm-peh-rah-<u>too</u>-rah)
toilet paper	el papel higiénico (ehl pah-<u>pehl</u> ee-<u>hyeh</u>-nēē-kaw)
tooth brush	el cepillo para dientes (ehl seh-<u>pēē</u>-yaw <u>pah</u>-rah <u>dyehn</u>-tehs)
toothpaste	pasta dentífrica (<u>pahs</u>-tah dehn-<u>tēē</u>-frēē-kah)
transfusion	la transfusión (lah trahns-foo-<u>syawn</u>)
urine	la orina (lah aw-<u>rēē</u>-nah)
(to) void	orinar (aw-r<u>ēē</u>-<u>nahr</u>)
(to) visit	visitar (b<u>ēē</u>-s<u>ēē</u>-<u>tahr</u>)
water	el agua (ehl <u>ah</u>-gwah)
- cold	fría (<u>frēē</u>-ah)
- hot	caliente (kah-<u>lyehn</u>-teh)
- iced	con hielo (kawn <u>yeh</u>-law)
- tepid	tibia (<u>tēē</u>-byah)

la silla
(lah see-yah)

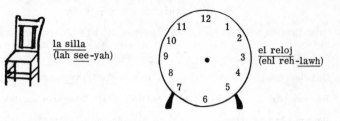
el reloj
(ehl reh-lawh)

la cama
(lah kah-mah)

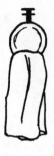
la toalla
(lah taw-ah-yah)

la taza de café
(lah tah-sah deh kah-feh)

el lavabo
(ehl lah-bah-baw)

el libro
(ehl lee-braw)

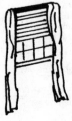
la ventana
(lah behn-tah-nah)

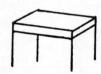
la mesa
(lah meh-sah)

un vaso de agua
(oon bah-saw deh ah-gwah)

CBB

THE LABORATORY TECHNICIAN

THE LABORATORY TECHNICIAN	EL TÉCNICO DEL LABORATORIO (ehl tehk-nee-kaw dehl lah-baw-rah-taw-ryaw)
Good morning!	¡Buenos días! (bweh-naw dee-ahs)
How are you?	¿Cómo está? (kaw-maw ehs-tah)
Have you had breakfast?	¿Se ha desayunado usted? (seh ah deh-sah-yoo-nah-daw oos-tehd)
I am going to take a blood sample.	Le voy a sacar una muestra de sangre. (leh bawy ah sah-kahr oo-nah mwehs-trah deh sahn-greh)
Relax! It will not hurt.	¡Relájese! No le va a doler. (reh-lah-heh-seh. naw leh bah ah daw-lehr)
Make a fist!	¡Haga un puño! (ah gah oon poon-yaw)
Open your hand!	¡Abra la mano! (ah-brah lah mah-naw)
Bend your elbow!	¡Doble el codo! (daw-bleh ehl kaw-daw)
Extend your index finger!	¡Extienda el índice! (ehgs-tyehn-dah ehl een-dee-seh)
This will feel like a slight pin prick.	Éste le parecerá como una pequeña picadura. (ehs-teh leh pah-reh-seh-rah kaw-maw oo-nah peh-kehn-yah pee-kah-doo-rah)
Please go to the bathroom and urinate in this receptacle.	Por favor, vaya al cuarto de baño y orine en este receptáculo. (pawr fah-bawr bah-yah ahl kwahr-taw deh bahn-yaw ee aw-ree-neh ehn ehs-teh reh-sehp-tah-koo-law)
I will need a stool specimen in this receptacle.	Necesito una nuestra de excremento en este receptáculo. (neh-seh-see-taw oo-nah mwehs-trah deh ehgs-kreh-mehn-taw ehn ehs-teh reh-sehp-tah-koo-law)
I have finished.	He terminado. (eh tehr-mee-nah-daw)
Thank you for your cooperation.	Gracias por su cooperación. (grah-syahs pawr soo kaw-aw-peh-rah-syawn

THE LABORATORY TECHNICIAN	EL TÉCNICO DEL LABORATORIO (ehl tehk-nee-kaw dehl lah-baw-rah-taw-ryaw)
Useful Vocabulary	Vocabulario Útil (baw-kah-boo-lah-ryaw oo-teel
albumin	la albumina (lah ahl-boo-mee-nah)
anaemia	la anemia (lah ah-neh-myah)
analysis	el análisis (ehl ah-nah-lee-sees)
arm	el brazo (ehl brah-saw)
bacteria	la bacteria (lah bahk-teh-ryah)
(to) bend	doblar (daw-blahr)
biopsy	la biopsia (lah bee-awp-syah)
(to) bleed	sangrar (sahn-grahr)
blood count	cuenta de glóbulos (kwehn-tah deh glaw-boo-laws)
blood sample	la muestra de sangre (lah mwehs-trah deh sahn-greh)
blood transfusion	la transfusión de sangre (lah trahns-foo-syawn deh sahn-greh)
diagnosis	la diagnosis (lah dee-ahg-naw-sees)
elbow	el codo (ehl kaw-daw)
finger	el dedo (ehl deh-daw)
- index	el índice (ehl een-dee-seh)
(to) finish	terminar (tehr-mee-nahr)
hand	la mano (lah mah-naw)
hemoglobin	la hemoglobina (lah eh-maw-glaw-bee-nah)
(to) hurt	doler (daw-lehr)
hypodermic needle	la aguja hipodérmica (lah ah-goo-hah ee-paw-dehr-mee-kah)
microbe	el microbio (ehl mee-kraw-byaw)
metabolism	el metabolismo (ehl meh-tah-baw-leez-maw)
pin prick	la picadura (lah pee-kah-doo-rah)
razor blade	la hoja de afeitar (lah aw-hah deh ah-fehy-tahr)

Relax!	¡Relájese! (reh-<u>lah</u>-heh-seh)
serum	el suero (ehl <u>sweh</u>-raw)
sputum	la esputa (lah ehs-<u>poo</u>-tah)
stool specimen	la muestra de excremento. (lah <u>mwehs</u>-trah deh ehgs-kreh-<u>mehn</u>-taw)
syringe	la jeringa (lah heh-<u>reen</u>-gah)
test	la prueba (lah <u>prweh</u>-bah)
thumb	el pulgar (ehl pool-<u>gahr</u>)
urine specimen	la muestra de orina (lah <u>mwehs</u>-trah deh aw-<u>ree</u>-nah)
vial	la ampolleta (lah ahm-paw-<u>yeh</u>-tah)
vomit	el vómito (ehl <u>baw</u>-<u>mee</u>-taw)

CCC

THE ANAESTHETIST

THE ANAESTHETIST	EL ANESTESISTA (ehl ah-neh-steh-<u>see</u>-stah)
Good morning!	¡Buenos días! (bweh-naws <u>dee</u>-ahs)
I am Dr. _____ .	Yo soy el doctor _____ . (yaw sawy ehl dawk-<u>tawr</u> _____).
I am going to administer the anaesthesia during your operation tomorrow.	Voy a darle la anestesia mañana durante la operación. (bawy ah <u>dahr</u>-leh lah ah-neh-steh-syah mahn-<u>yah</u>-nah doo-<u>rahn</u>-teh <u>lah</u> aw-peh-rah-<u>syawn</u>)
We need some pertinent information.	Necesitamos algunos datos pertinentes. (neh-seh-<u>see</u>-tah-maws ahl-<u>goo</u>-naws <u>dah</u>-taws pehr-<u>tee</u>-<u>nehn</u>-tehs)
Do you suffer from asthma, hay fever or allergies of any kind?	¿Sufre de asma, fiebre de heno o de alergias de alguna clase? (soo-freh deh <u>ahs</u>-mah, <u>fyeh</u>-breh deh eh-naw aw deh ah-<u>lehr</u>-hyahs deh ahl-<u>goo</u>-nah <u>klah</u>-seh)
When was your last attack and how bad was it?	¿Cuándo sufrió su último ataque y qué intensidad tuvo? (<u>kwahn</u>-daw soo-<u>fryaw</u> soo <u>ool</u>-<u>tee</u>-maw ah-<u>tah</u>-keh <u>ee</u> keh <u>een</u>-tehn-<u>see</u>-dahd <u>too</u>-baw)
Do you have a heart ailment?	¿Tiene enfermedad de corazón? (<u>tyeh</u>-neh ehn-fehr-meh-<u>dahd</u> deh kaw-rah-<u>sawn</u>)
Do you have any other chronic diseases?	¿Tiene algunas otras enfermedades crónicas? (<u>tyeh</u>-neh ahl-<u>goo</u>-nahs <u>aw</u>-trahs ehn-<u>fehr</u>-meh-<u>dah</u>-dehs <u>kraw</u>-<u>nee</u>-kahs)
Do you have high or low blood pressure?	¿Tiene la presión de sangre alta o baja? (<u>tyeh</u>-neh lah preh-<u>syawn</u> deh <u>sahn</u>-greh <u>ahl</u>-tah aw <u>bah</u>-hah)
Do you take any medicines? Which?	¿Toma usted algunas medicinas? ¿Cuáles? (<u>taw</u>-mah oos-tehd ahl-<u>goo</u>-nahs meh-<u>dee</u>-<u>see</u>-nahs. <u>kwah</u>-lehs)
Have you been operated before?	¿Ha sido operado antes? (ah <u>see</u>-daw aw-peh-<u>rah</u>-daw <u>ahn</u>-tehs)
When? What type of operation was it?	¿Cuándo? ¿Qué clase de operación fue? (<u>kwahn</u>-daw. keh <u>klah</u>-seh deh aw-peh-rah-<u>syawn</u> fweh)

Do you have a cold or sore throat?

¿Tiene catarro (resfriado) o dolor de garganta? (tyeh-neh kah-tahr-raw [rehs-free-ah-daw] aw daw-lawr deh gahr-gahn-tah)

Do you have a cough with much mucous?

¿Tiene tos con mucha flema? (tyeh-neh taws kawn moo-chah fleh-mah)

Do you smoke cigarettes? How many per day?

¿Fuma cigarrillos? ¿Cuántos por día? (foo-mah see-gahr-ree-yaws. kwahn-taws pawr dee-ah)

Are you taking any drugs or medicines? Which?

¿Está tomando algunas drogas o medicinas? ¿Cuáles? (ehs-tah taw-mahn-daw ahl-goo-nahs draw-gahs aw meh-dee-see-nahs. kwah-lehs)

We are going to give you a spinal injection.

Vamos a darle una inyección espinal. (bah-maws ah dahr-leh oo-nah een-yehk-syawn ehs-pee-nahl)

You will not feel any pain.

No sentirá ningún dolor. (naw sehn-tee-rah neen-goon daw-lawr)

You will receive a separate bill for the anaesthesia.

Para la anestesia usted recibirá una cuenta aparte de las otras. (pah-rah lah ah-nehs-teh-syah oos-tehd reh-see-bee-rah oo-nah kwehn-tah ah-pahr-teh deh lahs aw-trahs)

Everything is going to be fine.

Todo va a salir bien. (taw-daw bah ah sah-leer byehn)

BEFORE THE OPERATION

ANTES DE LA OPERACIÓN (ahn-tehs deh lah aw-peh-rah-syawn)

Have you had anything to eat or drink since midnight?

¿Ha tomado algo desde la medianoche? (ah taw-mah-daw ahl-gaw dehz-deh lah meh-dyah-naw-cheh)

Do you have dentures?

¿Tiene dentaduras? (tyeh-neh dehn-tah-doo-rahs)

Please remove them!

¡Quíteselos, por favor! (kee-teh-seh-laws, pawr fah-bawr)

Do you have chewing gum in your mouth?

¿Tiene chicle en la boca? (tyeh-neh chee-kleh ehn lah baw-kah)

Please take it out of your mouth.

Favor de sacarlo de la boca. (fah-bawr deh sah-kahr-law deh lah baw-kah)

Are you nauseous?

¿Tiene náusea? (tyeh-neh nah-oo-seh-ah)

Please move over to the table-bed.

Favor de moverse a la mesa cama. (fah-bawr deh maw-behr-seh ah lah meh-sah kah-mah)

Don't be afraid.   Everything is going to be all right.

No tenga miedo.   Todo va a salir muy bien.   (naw tehn-gah myeh-daw. taw-daw bah ah sah-leer mwee byehn)

Lie on your right (left) side.

Acuéstese sobre el lado derecho (izquierdo).   (ah-kweh-steh-seh saw-breh ehl lah-daw deh-reh-chaw [ees-kyehr-daw])

Draw up your knees.

Tire las rodillas hacia arriba. (tee-reh lahs raw-dee-yahs ah-syah ah-ree-bah)

We are going to give you an injection in the spine so that you will not feel any pain.

Vamos a darle una inyección en la espina dorsal para que no sienta ningún dolor.   (bah-maws ah dahr-leh oo-nah een-yehk-syawn ehn lah ehs-pee-nah dawr-sahl pah-rah keh naw syehn-tah neen-goon daw-lawr)

You will feel only a prick and then nothing more.

Va a sentir solamente una picadura y después nada más.   (bah ah sehn-teer saw-lah-mehn-teh oo-nah pee-kah-doo-rah ee dehs-pwehs nah-dah mahs)

THE ANAESTHETIST

EL ANESTESISTA (ehl ah-nehs-teh-see-stah)

Useful Vocabulary

Vocabulario Útil (baw-kah-boo-lah-ryaw oo-teel)

afraid

Tener miedo; temer   (teh-nehr myeh-daw; teh-mehr)

ailment

la enfermedad   (lah ehn-fehr-meh-dahd)

allergy

la alergia   (lah ah-lehr-hyah)

anaesthesia

la anestesia   (lah ah-nehs-teh-syah)

  - general

general   (heh-neh-rahl)

  - local

local   (law-kahl)

asthma

el asma   (ehl ahz-mah)

attack

el ataque   (ehl ah-tah-keh)

bill

la cuenta   (lah kwehn-tah)

blood pressure	la presión (lah preh-<u>syawn</u>)
- high	alta (<u>ahl</u>-tah)
- low	baja (<u>bah</u>-hah)
(to) breathe	respirar (rehs-p<u>ee</u>-<u>rahr</u>)
breathing	la respiración (lah rehs-p<u>ee</u>-rah- syawn)
chronic disease	la enfermedad crónica (lah ehn-fehr- meh-<u>dahd</u> <u>kraw</u>-n<u>ee</u>-kah)
cigarettes	los cigarillos (laws s<u>ee</u>-gah-r<u>ee</u>- yaws)
cold (to have a)	tener catarro; resfriado (teh-<u>nehr</u> kah-<u>tah</u>-raw; rehs-fr<u>ee</u>-ah-d<u>aw</u>)
condition	la condición (lah kawn-d<u>ee</u>-<u>syawn</u>)
cough	la tos (lah taws)
(to) cough	toser (taw-<u>sehr</u>)
Count up to 10 -- slowly!	¡Cuente hasta diez -- despacio! (<u>kwehn</u>-teh <u>ahs</u>-tah dyehs -- dehs- <u>pah</u>-syaw)
dentures	la dentadura (lah dehn-tah-<u>doo</u>-rah)
Don't be afraid!	¡No tenga miedo! (naw <u>tehn</u>-gah <u>myeh</u>-daw)
drugs	las drogas (lahs <u>draw</u>-gahs)
ether	el éter (ehl <u>eh</u>-tehr)
(to) feel pain	sentir dolor (sehn-t<u>eer</u> daw-<u>lawr</u>)
hay fever	la fiebre de heno (lah <u>fyeh</u>-breh deh <u>eh</u>-naw)
heart disease	la enfermedad de corazón (lah ehn- fehr-meh-<u>dahd</u> deh kaw-rah-<u>sawn</u>)
heart attack	el ataque al corazón (ehl ah-<u>tah</u>-keh ahl kaw-rah-<u>sawn</u>)
information	la información (lah <u>een</u>-fawr-mah- syawn)
injection	la inyección (lah <u>een</u>-yehk-<u>syawn</u>)
intensity	la intensidad (lah <u>een</u>-tehn-s<u>ee</u>- dahd)
Lie down!	¡Acuéstese! (ah-<u>kweh</u>-steh-seh)

left side	el lado izquierdo (ehl lah-daw ēēs-kyehr-daw)
mouth	la boca (lah baw-kah)
(to) move	moverse; trasladarse (maw-behr-seh; trahs-lah-dahr-seh)
nausea	la náusea (lah nah-oo-seh-ah)
(to be) nauseous	tener náusea (teh-nehr nah-oo-seh-ah)
(to) operate	operar (aw-peh-rahr)
operating room	la sala de operaciones (lah sah-lah deh aw-peh-rah-syaw-nehs)
operation	la operación (lah aw-peh-rah-syawn)
pain	el dolor (ehl daw-lawr)
prick	la picadura (lah pēē-kah-doo-rah)
(to) remove	quitar (kēē-tahr)
right side	el lado derecho (ehl lah-daw deh-reh-chaw)
Sit up!	¡Incorpórese! (ēēn-kawr-paw-reh-seh)
(to) smoke	fumar (foo-mahr)
spine	la espina dorsal (lah ehs-pēē-nah dawr-sahl)
suffer	sufrir (soo-frēēr)
tablebed	la mesa cama (lah meh-sah kah-mah)
(to) take out	sacar (sah-kahr)

ᏰᏰᏰ

THE GYNECOLOGIST

INTERVIEW WITH THE GYNECOLOGIST	ENTREVISTA CON EL GINECÓLOGO (ehn-treh-bēēs-tah kawn ehl hēē-neh-kaw-law-gaw)
What is your name?	¿Cómo se llama usted? (kaw-maw seh yah-mah oos-tehd)
How old are you?	¿Qué edad tiene usted? (keh eh-dahd tyeh-neh oos-tehd)
Do you work outside the home?	¿Trabaja fuera de la casa? (trah-bah-hah fweh-rah deh lah kah-sah)
What kind of work do you do?	¿Qué clase de trabajo hace usted? (keh klah-seh deh trah-bah-haw ah-seh oos-tehd)
What is your religion?	¿Cuál es su religión? (kwahl ehs soo reh-lēē-hyawn)
At what age did you begin to menstruate?	¿A qué edad empezó usted a menstruar? (ah keh eh-dahd ehm-peh-saw oos-tehd ah mehn-stroo-ahr)
Are your menstrual periods regular or irregular? Explain.	¿Son sus menstruos regulares o irregulares? Explique usted. (sawn soos mehn-stroo-aws reh-goo-lah-rehs aw ēē-reh-goo-lah-rehs. ehks-plēē-keh oos-tehd)
How many days does each period last?	¿Cuántos días dura cada periodo? (kwahn-taws dēē-ahs doo-rah cah-dah peh-ryaw-daw)
Does the blood flow freely or is it coagulated?	¿Corre libremente la sangre, o está coagulada? (kaw-reh lēē-breh-mehn-teh lah sahn-greh aw ehs-tah kaw-ah-goo-lah-dah)
Do you bleed outside of your period?	¿Sangra usted fuera de su periodo? (sahn-grah oos-tehd fweh-rah deh soo peh-ryaw-daw)
Do you bleed after intercourse?	¿Sangra usted después del coito? (sahn-grah oos-tehd dehs-pwehs dehl kawy-taw)
Do you have any pain at the time of menstruation?	¿Sufre usted algunos dolores durante algún tiempo del periodo? (soo-freh oos-tehd ahl-goo-naws daw-law-rehs doo-rahn-teh ahl-goon tyehm-po dehl peh-ryaw-daw)

- Before?

¿Antes? (ahn-tehs)

- During?

¿Mientras que menstrua? (myehn-trahs keh mehn-stroo-ah)

- After?

¿Después? (dehs-pwehs)

Do you have any difficulty urinating?

¿Tiene usted alguna dificultad en orinar? (tyeh-neh oos-tehd ahl-goo-nah dee-fee-kool-tahd ehn aw-ree-nahr)

Do you have any allergies?

¿Sufre usted de algunas alergias? (soo-freh oos-tehd deh ahl-goo-nahs ah-lehr-hyahs)

Do you take any medicines? Which?

¿Toma usted algunas medicinas? ¿Cuáles? (taw-mah oos-tehd ahl-goo-nahs meh-dee-see-nahs. kwah-lehs)

Is this your first pregnancy?

¿Es éste su primer embarazo? (ehs ehs-teh soo pree-mehr ehm-bah-rah-saw)

Have you had any miscarriages?

¿Ha tenido usted algunos abortos espontáneos? (ah teh-nee-daw oos-tehd ahl-goo-naws ah-bawr-taws ehs-pawn-tah-neh-aws)

Have you had any still births?

¿Ha tenido usted alguna criatura que haya nacido muerta? (ah teh-nee-daw oos-tehd ahl-goo-nah kree-ah-too-rah keh ah-yah nah-see-daw mwehr-tah)

Have you had any abnormal pregnancies outside the uterus (ectopic pregnancies), or in the Fallopian tubes?

¿Ha tenido usted algún embarazo anormal fuera de la matriz (embarazos ectópicos), o en las trompas de Falopio? (ah teh-nee-daw oos-tehd ahl-goon ehm-bah-rah-saw ah-nawr-mahl fweh-rah deh lah mah-trees [ehm-bah-rah-saws ehk-taw-pee-kaws] aw ehn lahs trawm-pahs deh fah-law-pyaw)

Have you used any kind of contraceptive?

¿Ha usado usted contraceptivos de alguna clase? (ah oo-sah-daw oos-tehd kawn-trah-sehp-tee-baws deh ahl-goo-nah klah-seh)

- the pill?

¿la píldora? (lah peel-daw-rah)

- condom?

¿el condón? (ehl kawn-dawn)

- diaphragm?

¿el diafragma? (ehl dee-ah-frahg-mah)

- douches?

¿duchas? (doo-chahs)

- suppositories?

¿ supositorios? (soo-paw-s<u>ee</u>-taw-ryaws)

- foam?

¿ medicinas espumosas? (meh-d<u>ee</u>-s<u>ee</u>-nahs ehs-poo-<u>maw</u>-sahs)

Have you ever had syphilis or gonorrhea?

¿ Ha tenido usted alguna vez sífilis o gonorrea? (ah teh-n<u>ee</u>-daw oos-tehd ahl-<u>goo</u>-nah vehs s<u>ee</u>-f<u>ee</u>-l<u>ees</u> aw gaw-naw-<u>reh</u>-ah)

Were you treated for them?

¿ Tuvo usted tratamiento para ellos? (<u>too</u>-baw oos-tehd trah-tah-<u>myehn</u>-taw <u>pah</u>-rah <u>eh</u>-yaws)

Have you had any other venereal diseases?

¿ Ha tenido usted alguna otra clase de enfermedad venérea? (ah teh-n<u>ee</u>-daw oos-<u>tehd</u> ahl-<u>goo</u>-nah aw-trah klah-seh <u>deh</u> ehn-<u>fehr</u>-meh-dahd <u>beh</u>-<u>neh</u>-reh-ah)

Do you have diabetes?

¿ Tiene usted diabetes? (<u>tyeh</u>-neh oos-<u>tehd</u> d<u>ee</u>-ah-<u>beh</u>-tehs)

Do you use drugs of any kind?

¿ Usa usted drogas de alguna clase? (oo-sah oos-tehd <u>draw</u>-gahs deh ah<u>l</u>-<u>goo</u>-nah <u>klah</u>-seh)

Have you ever had any blood transfusions?

¿ Ha tenido jamás algunas transfusiones de sangre? (ah teh-n<u>ee</u>-daw hah-<u>mahs</u> ahl-<u>goo</u>-nahs trahns-foo-<u>syaw</u>-nehs deh <u>sahn</u>-greh)

What blood type do you have?

¿ Qué clasificación de sangre tiene? (keh klah-s<u>ee</u>-f<u>ee</u>-kah-<u>syawn</u> deh sahn-greh <u>tyeh</u>-neh)

You have varicose veins.

Usted tiene venas varicosas. (oos-tehd <u>tyeh</u>-neh <u>beh</u>-nahs bah-<u>ree</u>-<u>kaw</u>-sahs)

I am going to examine you through the vagina and the rectum. It will not hurt you.

Voy a examinarla por la vagina y por el recto. No le va a doler. (bawy ah ehgs-ah-m<u>ee</u>-<u>nahr</u>-lah pawr lah bah-<u>hee</u>-nah <u>ee</u> pawr ehl <u>rehk</u>-taw. naw <u>leh</u> bah ah daw-<u>lehr</u>)

Your pelvis is too narrow for the baby to be born through the vagina.

La pelvis es demasiado estrecha para que el bebé nazca por la vagina. (lah <u>pehl</u>-b<u>ees</u> ehs deh-mah-<u>syah</u>-daw ehs-<u>treh</u>-chah <u>pah</u>-rah keh ehl beh-<u>beh</u> <u>nahs</u>-kah pawr lah bah-<u>hee</u>-nah)

You will need a Caesarean operation.

Necesitará una operación cesárea. (neh-seh-s<u>ee</u>-tah-rah oo-nah aw-peh-rah-<u>syawn</u> seh-<u>sah</u>-reh-ah)

We shall have to terminate the pregnancy.	Tenemos que terminar el embarazo. (teh-<u>neh</u>-maws keh tehr-m<u>ee</u>-nahr ehl e<u>hm</u>-bah-<u>rah</u>-saw)
You will need a hysterectomy.	Necesitará una operación uterina. (neh-seh-s<u>ee</u>-tah-<u>rah</u> oo-nah aw-peh-rah-<u>syawn</u> oo-teh-<u>ree</u>-nah)

INTERVIEW WITH THE
  GYNECOLOGIST

ENTREVISTA CON EL
  GINECÓLOGO
(ehn-treh-b<u>ees</u>-tah kawn ehl h<u>ee</u>-neh-kaw-<u>law</u>-gaw)

Useful Vocabulary	Vocabulario Útil (baw-kah-boo-<u>lah</u>-ryaw oo-t<u>ee</u>l)
abnormal	anormal (ah-nawr-<u>mahl</u>)
abortion	el aborto (ehl ah-<u>bawr</u>-taw)
age	la edad (lah eh-<u>dahd</u>)
allergy	la alergia (lah ah-<u>lehr</u>-hyah)
appointment	la cita (lah s<u>ee</u>-tah)
baby	el bebé, la criatura (ehl beh-<u>beh</u>. lah kr<u>ee</u>-ah-<u>too</u>-rah)
bath	el baño (ehl <u>bahn</u>-yaw)
- tepid	tibio (t<u>ee</u>-byaw)
- hot	caliente (kah-<u>lyehn</u>-teh)
- cold	frío (fr<u>ee</u>-aw)
(to) begin	empezar (ehm-peh-<u>sahr</u>)
bladder	la vejiga (lah beh-h<u>ee</u>-gah)
(to) bleed	sangrar (sahn-<u>grahr</u>)
blood count	la cuenta de glóbulos (lah kwehn-tah deh <u>glaw</u>-boo-laws)
blood pressure	la presión de la sangre (lah preh-<u>syawn</u> deh lah <u>sahn</u>-greh)
- high	alta (<u>ahl</u>-tah)
- low	baja (<u>bah</u>-hah)
breast	el pecho (ehl <u>peh</u>-chaw)
Caesarean operation	la operación cesárea (lah aw-peh-rah-<u>syawn</u> seh-<u>sah</u>-reh-ah)
coagulated blood	la sangre coagulada (lah <u>sahn</u>-greh kaw-ah-goo-<u>lah</u>-dah)

coitus	el coito (ehl <u>kawy</u>-taw)
condom	el condón (ehl kawn-<u>dawn</u>)
consultation	la consulta (lah kawn-<u>sool</u>-tah)
contraceptive	el contraceptivo (ehl kawn-trah-sehp-<u>tee</u>-baw)
(to) cure	curar (koo-<u>rahr</u>)
daily	por día (pawr <u>dee</u>-ah)
day	el día (ehl <u>dee</u>-ah)
diabetes	diabetes (<u>dee</u>-ah-<u>beh</u>-tehs)
difficulty	la dificultad (lah <u>dee</u>-fee-kool-<u>tahd</u>)
douche	la ducha (lah <u>doo</u>-chah)
drugs	las drogas (lahs <u>draw</u>-gahs)
embryo	el embrión (ehl ehm-<u>bryawn</u>)
examine	examinar; investigar (ehgs-ah-<u>mee</u>-nahr; <u>een</u>-behs-tee-<u>gahr</u>)
Fallopian tubes	las trompas de Falopio (lahs <u>trawm</u>-pahs deh fah-<u>law</u>-pyaw)
foetus	el feto (ehl <u>feh</u>-taw)
(to) flow	derramar (deh-rah-<u>mahr</u>)
foam (contraceptive)	la medicina espumosa (lah meh-<u>dee</u>-<u>see</u>-nah ehs-poo-<u>maw</u>-sah)
gonorrhea	gonorrea (gaw-naw-<u>reh</u>-ah)
gynecologist	el ginecólogo (ehl <u>gee</u>-neh-<u>kaw</u>-law-gaw)
(to) hurt (someone)	hacer daño a (ah-<u>sehr</u> <u>dahn</u>-yaw ah)
hysterectomy	la operación uterina (lah aw-peh-rah-<u>syawn</u> oo-teh-<u>ree</u>-nah)
hemorrhage	la hemorragia (lah eh-maw-<u>rah</u>-hyah)
hereditary	hereditario (eh-reh-dee-<u>tah</u>-ryaw)
illegitimate	ilegítimo (masculine) (<u>ee</u>-leh-<u>hee</u>-<u>tee</u>-maw) ilegítima (feminine) (<u>ee</u>-leh-<u>hee</u>-<u>tee</u>-mah)
intercourse (sexual)	el coito; las relaciones sexuales (ehl <u>kawy</u>-taw; lahs reh-lah-<u>syaw</u>-nehs <u>sehgs</u>-<u>wah</u>-lehs)

interview	la entrevista (lah ehn-treh-b<u>ee</u>s-tah)
irregular	irregular (<u>ee</u>r-reh-goo-<u>lahr</u>)
(to) last	durar (doo-<u>rahr</u>)
labor pains	dolores de parto (daw-<u>law</u>-rehs deh <u>pahr</u>-taw)
measles	el sarampión (ehl sah-rahm-<u>pyawn</u>)
- German measles	la rubéola (lah roo-<u>beh</u>-aw-lah)
medicine	la medicina (lah meh-d<u>ee</u>-s<u>ee</u>-nah)
(to) menstruate	menstruar (mehn-stroo-<u>ahr</u>)
menopause	la menopausia (lah meh-naw-<u>pah</u>-oo-syah)
menstruation	la menstruación (lah mehn-stroo-ah-<u>syawn</u>)
miscarriage	el aborto espontáneo (ehl ah-<u>bawr</u>-taw ehs-pawn-<u>tah</u>-neh-aw)
morning sickness	los vómitos de embarazo (laws baw-m<u>ee</u>-taws deh ehm-bah-<u>rah</u>-saw)
name	el nombre (ehl <u>nawm</u>-breh)
narrow	estrecho (masculine) (ehs-<u>treh</u>-chaw) estrecha (feminine) (ehs-<u>treh</u>-chah)
nipple (breast)	el pezón (ehl peh-<u>sawn</u>)
nurse	la enfermera (lah ehn-fehr-<u>meh</u>-rah)
(to) operate	operar (aw-peh-<u>rahr</u>)
operation	la operación (lah aw-peh-rah-<u>syawn</u>)
ovaries	los ovarios (laws aw-<u>bah</u>-ryaws)
pain	el dolor (ehl daw-<u>lawr</u>)
pelvis	la pelvis (lah <u>pehl</u>-b<u>ee</u>s)
pessary	el pesario (ehl peh-<u>sah</u>-ryaw)
pill	la píldora (lah p<u>eel</u>-daw-rah)
pregnancy	el embarazo (ehl ehm-bah-<u>rah</u>-saw)
rectum	el recto (ehl <u>rehk</u>-taw)
regular	regular (reh-goo-<u>lahr</u>)

religion	la religión (lah reh-lee-hyawn)
RH factor	el factor Rhesus (ehl fahk-tawr reh-soos)
sexual relations	las relaciones sexuales (lahs reh-lah-syaw-nehs sehgs-wah-lehs)
stillborn	nacido muerto (nah-see-daw mwehr-taw)
(to) suffer	sufrir (soo-freer)
suppository	el supositorio (ehl soo-paw-see-taw-ryaw)
syphilis	sífilis (see-fee-lees)
treatment	el tratamiento (ehl trah-tah-myehn-taw)
transfusion	la transfusión (lah trahns-foo-syawn)
urinate	orinar (aw-ree-nahr)
uterus	el útero; la matriz (ehl oo-teh-raw; lah mah-trees)
vagina	la vagina (lah bah-hee-nah)
varicose veins	las venas varicosas (lahs beh-nahs bah-ree-kaw-sahs)
venereal disease	la enfermedad venérea (lah ehn-fehr-meh-dahd beh-neh-reh-ah)
womb	el útero; la matriz (ehl oo-teh-raw; lah mah-trees)

THE PSYCHIATRIST

INTERVIEW WITH THE PSYCHIATRIST	ENTREVISTA CON EL PSIQUIATRA (ehn-treh-bee-stah kawn ehl see-kyah-trah)
What is your name?	¿Cuál es su nombre? (kwahl ehs soo nawm-breh)
What is your address?	¿Cuál es su dirección? (kwahl ehs soo dee-rehk-syawn)
What is your telephone number?	¿Cuál es su número de teléfono? (kwahl ehs soo noo-meh-raw deh teh-leh-faw-naw)
What is your social security number?	¿Cuál es su número de seguro social? (kwahl ehs soo noo-meh-raw deh seh-goo-raw saw-syahl)
What is your religion?	¿Cuál es su religión? (kwahl ehs soo reh-lee-hyawn)
What profession do you practice?	¿Cuál es su profesión? (kwahl ehs soo praw-feh-syawn)
What is your problem?	¿Cuál es su problema? (kwahl ehs soo praw-bleh-mah)
	¿De qué se queja usted? (deh keh seh keh-hah oos-tehd)
What are your symptoms?	¿Cuáles son sus síntomas? (kwah-lehs sawn soos seen-taw-mahs)
Is there anyone in your family who has had any mental illnesses or of the nervous system?	¿Hay alguien en su familia que haya sufrido de enfermedades mentales o del sistema nervioso? (ahy ahl-gyehn ehn soo fah-mee-lyah keh ah-yah soo-free-daw deh ehn-fehr-meh-dah-dehs mehn-tah-lehs aw dehl sees-teh-mah nehr-byaw-saw)
What type of work do you do?	¿Qué clase de trabajo hace usted? (keh klah-seh deh trah-bah-haw ah-seh oos-tehd)
Are you exposed to toxic material during your work?	¿Está expuesto a materias tóxicas durante el trabajo? (ehs-tah ehgs-pweh-staw ah mah-teh-ryahs tawk-see-kahs doo-rahn-teh ehl trah-bah-haw)
Do you have difficulties with your co-workers?	¿Tiene dificultades con sus compañeros de trabajo? (tyeh-neh dee-fee-kool-tah-dehs kawn soos kawm-pahn-yeh-raws deh trah-bah-haw)

Do you have family problems?	¿Tiene problemas con su familia? (tyeh-neh praw-bleh-mahs kawn soo fah-meel-yah)
Do you have recurrent fears?	¿Tiene usted miedos que recurran frecuentemente? (tyeh-neh oos-tehd myeh-daws keh reh-koo-rahn freh-kwehn-teh-mehn-teh)
Do you fear that everyone wants to harm you?	¿Tiene miedos que todo el mundo quiera hacerle daño? (tyeh-neh myeh-daws keh taw-daw ehl moon-daw kyeh- rah ah-sehr-leh dahn-yaw)
How long have you had these fears?	¿Desde cuándo tiene usted estos miedos? dehz-deh kwahn-daw tyeh-neh oos-tehd ehs-taws myeh-daws)
Do you use drugs or sedatives of any kind?	¿Usa usted drogas o sedativos de alguna clase? (oo-sah oos-tehd draw-gahs aw seh-dah-tee-baws deh ahl-goo-nah klah-seh)
Do you take alcoholic beverages? How much?	¿Toma usted bebidas alcohólicas? ¿Cuántas? (taw-mah oos-tehd beh-bee-dahs al-kaw-aw-lee-kahs. kwahn tas)
Do you smoke? How much?	¿Fuma usted? Cuánto? (foo-mah oos-tehd. kwahn-taw)
Have you had any venereal diseases?	¿Ha tenido usted alguna enfermedad venérea? (ah teh-nee-daw oos-tehd ahl-goo-nah ehn-fehr-meh-dahd beh-neh-reh-ah)
- Syphilis?	¿Sífilis? (see-fee-lees)
- Gonorrhea?	¿Gonorrea? (gaw-naw-reh-ah)
Do you suffer from insomnia?	¿Sufre usted de insomnio? (soo-freh oos-tehd deh een-sawm-nyaw)
Do you have many worries, responsibilities, debts?	¿Tiene muchas preocupaciones, responsabilidades, deudas? (tyeh-neh oos-tehd moo-chahs preh-aw-koo-pah-syaw-nehs, rehs-pawn-sah-bee-lee-dah-dehs, deh-oo-dahs)
Do you take regular vacations?	¿Va de vacaciones regularmente? (bah deh bah-kah-syaw-nehs reh-goo-lahr-mehn-teh)
Come to see me next week.	Venga a verme la semana próxima. (behn-gah ah behr-meh lah seh-mah-nah prawk-see-mah)

INTERVIEW WITH THE PSYCHIATRIST	ENTREVISTA CON EL PSICHIATRA (ehn-treh-bēē-stah kawn ehl sēē-kyah-trah)
Useful Vocabulary	Vocabulario Útil (baw-kah-boo-lah-ryaw oo-tēēl)
addict	el adicto (ehl ah-dēēk-taw)
address	la dirección (lah dēē-rehk-syawn)
alcoholic	el alcohólico (ehl ahl-kaw-aw-lēē-kaw)
arteriosclerosis	arterio-esclerosis (ahr-teh-ryaw-ehs-kleh-raw-sēēs)
(to) calm	calmar (kahl-mahr)
complain	quejarse (keh-hahr-seh)
complaint	la queja (lah keh-hah)
delusion	la delusión (lah deh-loo-syawn)
dementia	la dimencia (lah dēē-mehn-syah)
depression	la depresión (lah deh-preh-syawn)
(to) drink	beber (beh-behr)
drugs	las drogas (lahs draw-gahs)
fear	el miedo (ehl myeh-daw)
(to) fear	tener miedo; temer (teh-nehr myeh-daw; teh-mehr)
gonorrhea	gonorrea (gaw-naw-reh-ah)
hallucination	la halucinación (lah ah-loo-sēē-nah-syawn)
head	la cabeza (lah kah-beh-sah)
(to) hear	oír (aw-ēēr)
hysteria	la histeria (lah ēēs-teh-ryah)
idiocy	la idiotez (lah ēē-dyaw-tehs)
idiot	idiota (ēē-dyaw-tah)
injection	la inyección (lah ēēn-yehk-syawn)
insanity	la locura (lah law-koo-rah)
masturbation	masturbación (mahs-toor-bah-syawn)

mental illness	la enfermedad mental (lah ehn-fehr-meh-<u>dahd</u> mehn-<u>tahl</u>)
name	el nombre (ęhl <u>nawm</u>-breh)
nerves	los nervios (laws <u>nehr</u>-byaws)
nervous breakdown	la crisis nerviosa (lah <u>krēē</u>-sēēs nehr-<u>byaw</u>-sah)
nightmare	la pesadilla (lah peh-sah-<u>dēē</u>-yah)
nurse	la enfermera (lah ehn-fehr-<u>meh</u>-rah)
paranoia	paranoia (pah-rah-<u>naw</u>-yah)
patient	el paciente (masculine) (ehl pah-<u>syehn</u>-teh) la paciente (feminine) (lah pah-<u>syehn</u>-teh)
personality	la personalidad (lah pehr-saw-nah-<u>lēē</u>-dahd)
psychiatry	la psichiatría (lah sēē-kyah-<u>trēē</u>-yah)
psychoanalysis	psicoanálisis (sēē-kaw-ah-<u>nah</u>-<u>lēē</u>-sēēs)
psychopath	psicópata (sēē-<u>kaw</u>-pah-tah)
psychosis	psicosis (sēē-<u>kaw</u>-sēēs)
restlessness	la inquietud (lah ēēn-kyeh-<u>tood</u>)
sedative	el sedativo (ehl seh-dah-<u>tēē</u>-baw)
(to) smoke	fumar (foo-<u>mahr</u>)
symptoms	los síntomas (laws <u>sēēn</u>-taw-mahs)
tranquilizer	el calmante (ehl kahl-<u>mahn</u>-teh)
venereal disease	la enfermedad venérea (lah ehn-fehr-meh-<u>dahd</u> beh-<u>neh</u>-reh-ah)
voices	las voces (lahs <u>baw</u>-sehs)
schizophrenia	la esquizofrenia (lah ehs-kēē-saw-<u>freh</u>-nyah)

GGG

HEART AND LUNGS

HEART AND LUNGS	EL CORAZÓN Y LOS PULMONES (ehl kaw-rah-<u>sawn</u> <u>ee</u> laws pool-<u>maw</u>-nehs)
Do you have shortness of breath?	¿Le falta aliento? ¿Cuándo? (leh <u>fahl</u>-tah ah-<u>lyehn</u>-taw. <u>kwahn</u>-daw)
Do you have fainting spells?	¿Tiene usted ataques de desvanecimiento? (<u>tyeh</u>-neh oos-<u>tehd</u> ah-<u>tah</u>-kehs deh <u>dehs</u>-bah-neh-<u>see</u>-myehn-taw)
When did they start? How often do you have them?	¿Cuándo empezaron? ¿Cuántas veces? (<u>kwahn</u>-daw ehm-peh-<u>sah</u>-rawn. <u>kwahn</u>-tahs beh-sehs)
Do you have dizzy spells? How often?	¿Tiene usted ataques de vértigo? ¿Cuántas veces? (<u>tyeh</u>-neh oos-tehd ah-<u>tah</u>-kehs deh <u>behr-tee</u>-gaw. <u>kwahn</u>-tahs beh-sehs)
Do you suffer from pains in your chest?	¿Sufre usted de dolores de pecho? (<u>soo</u>-freh oos-<u>tehd</u> deh daw-<u>law</u>-rehs deh <u>peh</u>-chaw)
Do you suffer from headaches?	¿Sufre usted de dolores de cabeza? (<u>soo</u>-freh oos-<u>tehd</u> deh daw-<u>law</u>-rehs deh kah-<u>beh</u>-sah)
Do you cough much?	¿Tose usted mucho? (<u>taw</u>-seh oos-tehd <u>moo</u>-chaw)
When you expectorate is there blood in the sputum?	Cuando expectora ¿hay sangre en el esputo? (<u>kwahn</u>-daw ehgs-pehk-<u>taw</u>-rah ahy <u>sahn</u>-greh ehn ehl ehs-<u>poo</u>-taw)
Have you had pneumonia?	¿Ha tenido usted pulmonía? (ah teh-<u>nee</u>-daw oos-<u>tehd</u> pool-maw-<u>nee</u>-ah)
- pleurisy?	¿pleuresía? (pleh-oo-reh-<u>see</u>-ah)
- bronchitis?	¿bronquitis? (brawn-<u>kee-tees</u>)
Do you smoke? How many cigarettes per day?	¿Fuma usted? ¿Cuántos cigarillos por día? (<u>foo</u>-mah oos-<u>tehd</u>. <u>kwahn</u>-taws <u>see</u>-gah-<u>ree</u>-yaws pawr <u>dee</u>-ah)
Does anyone in your family suffer from heart disease?	¿Hay alguien en su familia que sufra de enfermedad de corazón? (ahy <u>ahl</u>-ghyehn ehn soo fah-<u>meel</u>-yah <u>keh</u> soo-frah deh ehn-fehr-meh-<u>dahd</u> deh kaw-rah-<u>sawn</u>)

Does anyone in your family suffer from lung disease?	¿Hay alguien en su familia que sufra de enfermedad de pulmones? (ahy ahl-ghyehn ehn soo fah-meel-yah keh soo-frah deh ehn-fehr-meh-dahd deh pool-maw-nehs)
How many in your family have died from heart or lung disease?	¿Cuántos en su familia han muerto de enfermedades de corazón o de pulmones? (kwahn-taws ehn soo fah-meel-yah ahn mwehr-taw deh ehn-fehr-meh-dah-dehs deh kaw-rah-sawn aw deh pool-maw-nehs)
Do your ankles swell?	¿Se le hinchan los tobillos? (seh leh een-chahn laws taw-bee-yaws)
- During the day?	¿Por el día? (pawr ehl dee-ah)
- At night?	¿Por la noche? (pawr lah naw-cheh)
Do you have pains in your left arm at times?	¿Tiene dolores en el brazo izquierdo a veces? (tyeh-neh daw-law-rehs ehn ehl brah-saw ees-kyehr-daw ah beh-sehs)
Do you have palpitations of the heart?	¿Tiene usted palpitaciones del corazón? (tyeh-neh oos-tehd pahl-pee-tah-syaw-nehs dehl kaw-rah-sawn)
- Frequently?	¿Frecuentemente? (freh-kwehn-teh-mehn-teh)
- When?	¿Cuándo? (kwahn-daw)
Have you been treated for heart (or lung) disease before?	¿Ha sido tratado (tratada) para alguna enfermedad de corazón (o de pulmones) antes? (ah see-daw trah-tah-daw [trah-tah-dah] pah-rah ahl-goo-nah ehn-fehr-meh-dahd deh kaw-rah-sawn [aw deh pool-maw-nehs] ahn-tehs)
- When?	¿Cuándo (kwahn-daw)
- For how long?	¿Por cuánto tiempo? (pawr kwahn-taw tyehm-paw)
- By whom?	¿Por quién? (pawr kyehn)
Have you been treated for any other disease?	¿Ha sido tratado (tratada) para alguna otra enfermedad? (ah see-daw trah-tah-daw [trah-tah-dah] pah-rah ahl-goo-nah aw-trah ehn-fehr-meh-dahd)
Have you had rheumatic fever?	¿Ha tenido usted fiebre reumática? (ah teh-nee-daw oos-tehd fyeh-breh reh-oo-mah-tee-kah)

Do you have diabetes?

¿Tiene usted diabetes? (tyeh-neh oos-tehd dyah-beh-tehs)

Are you taking any drugs or medicines?

¿Está tomando algunas drogas o medicinas? (ehs-tah taw-mahn-daw ahl-goo-nahs draw-gahs aw meh-dee-see-nahs)

Do you take alcoholic beverages? How much?

¿Toma bebidas alcohólicas? ¿Cuántas? (taw-mah beh-bee-dahs ahl-kaw-aw-lee-kahs. kwahn-tahs)

Do you drink coffee or tea? How much?

¿Bebe usted café o té? ¿Cuánto? (beh-beh oos-tehd kah-feh aw teh. kwahn-taw)

You will have to spend a few days in the hospital. It will be necessary to make some tests.

Tiene que pasar algunos días en el hospital. Tenemos que hacer algunas investigaciones. (tyeh-neh keh pah-sahr ahl-goo-naws dee-ahs ehn ehl aws-pee-tahl. teh-neh-maws keh ah-sehr ahl-goo-nahs een-behs-tee-gah-syaw-nehs)

I shall give you a prescription.

Le daré una receta. (leh dah-reh oo-nah reh-seh-tah)

Take these pills three times a day, two after each meal.

Tome estas píldoras tres veces por día, dos después de cada comida. (taw-meh ehs-tahs peel-daw-rahs trehs beh-sehs pawr dee-ah, daws dehs-pwehs deh kah-dah kaw-mee-dah)

You must stay in bed for at least ten days.

Tiene que guardar cama por diez días, por lo menos. (tyeh-neh keh gwahr-dahr kah-mah pawr dyehs dee-ahs, pawr law meh-naws)

I shall examine you again at the end of ten days.

Le haré otro examen al final de los diez días. (leh ah-reh aw-traw ehg-sah-mehn ahl fee-nahl deh laws dyehs dee-ahs)

We shall have to take X-rays of your chest.

Tenemos que sacar rayos equis del pecho. (teh-neh-maws keh sah-kahr rah-yaws eh-kees dehl peh-chaw)

We will have to take an electro-cardiogram.

Tenemos que sacar un electro-cardiograma. (teh-neh-maws keh sah-kahr oon eh-lehk-traw kahr-dyaw-grah-mah)

We shall have to take some blood samples.

Tenemos que sacar muestras de sangre. (teh-neh-maws keh sah-kahr mwehs-trahs deh sahn-greh)

When the reports are completed, I shall get in touch with you.	Cuando las investigaciones estén completadas, le llamaré. (kwahn-daw lahs ēēn-behs-tēē-gah-syaw-nehs ehs-tehn kawm-pleh-tah-dahs, le yah-mah-reh)
HEART AND LUNGS	EL CORAZÓN Y LOS PULMONES (ehl kaw-rah-sawn ēē laws pool-maw-nehs)
Useful Vocabulary	Vocabulario Útil (baw-kah-boo-lah-ryaw oo-tēēl)
aneurism	la aneurisma (lah ah-neh-oo-rēēs-mah)
angina	la angina (lah ahn-hēē-nah)
ankles	los tobillos (laws taw-bēē-yaws)
arm	el brazo (ehl brah-saw)
arteriosclerosis	la arteriosclerosis (lah ahr-teh-ryaw-skleh-raw-sēēs)
asthma	asma (ahs-mah)
black-outs	momentos en que no se ve (maw-mehn-taws ehn keh naw seh beh)
blood pressure	la presión de sangre (lah preh-syawn deh sahn-greh)
- high	alta (ahl-tah)
- low	baja (bah-hah)
breath	el aliento; la respiración (ehl ah-lyehn-taw; lah rehs-pēē-rah-syawn)
- shortness of breath	cortedad de aliento (kawr-teh-dahd deh ah-lyehn-taw)
bronchitis	la bronquitis (lah brawn-kēē-tēēs)
chest	el pecho (ehl peh-chaw)
cigarettes	los cigarillos (laws sēē-gah-rēē-yaws)
clot	el coágulo (ehl kaw-ah-goo-law)
coffee	el café (ehl kah-feh)
coronary thrombosis	trombosis de la coronaria (trawm-baw-sēēs deh lah kaw-raw-nah-ryah)
cough	la tos (lah taws)

cold   el resfriado; el catarro (ehl rehs-
                                         free-ah-daw; ehl kah-tah-raw)

diabetes   la diabetes (lah dyah-beh-tehs)

diarrhea   la diarrea (lah dyah-reh-yah)

dizziness   el vértigo (ehl behr-tee-gaw)

drugs   las drogas (lahs draw-gahs)

electrocardiogram   el electrocardiograma (ehl eh-lehk-
                                         traw-kahr-dyaw-grah-mah)

(to) examine   examinar (ehg-sah-mee-nahr)

exhale   exhalar (ehg-sah-lahr)

expectorate   expectorar (ehgs-pehk-taw-rahr)

fainting   el desmayo (ehl dehs-mah-yaw)

(to) faint   desmayarse (dehs-mah-yahr-seh)

frequently   con frecuencia; frecuentemente
                                         (kawn freh-kwehn-syah; freh-kwehn-
                                         teh-mehn-teh)

headache   el dolor de cabeza (ehl daw-lawr
                                         deh kah-beh-sah)

heart disease   la enfermedad de corazón (lah ehn-
                                         fehr-meh-dahd deh kaw-rah-sawn)

hospital   el hospital (ehl aws-pee-tahl)

indigestion   la indigestión (lah een-dee-hehs-
                                         tyawn)

inhale   inhalar (een-ah-lahr)

injurious   dañoso (dahn-yaw-saw)

left side   el lado izquierdo (ehl lah-daw ees-
                                         kyehr-daw)

lungs   los pulmones (laws pool-maw-nehs)

(to be) necessary   ser necesario (sehr neh-seh-sah-
                                         ryaw)

nurse   la enfermera (lah ehn-fehr-meh-
                                         rah)

obesity   el sobrepeso (ehl saw-breh-peh-
                                         saw)

obstruction   la obstrucción (lah awb-strook-
                                         syawn)

pain	el dolor (ehl daw-<u>lawr</u>)
- sharp	agudo (ah-<u>goo</u>-daw)
palpitation	la palpitación (lah pahl-p<u>ee</u>-tah- <u>syawn</u>)
paralysis	la parálisis (lah pah-<u>rah</u>-l<u>ee</u>-s<u>ee</u>s)
phlegm	las flemas (lahs <u>fleh</u>-mahs)
pleurisy	la pleuresía (lah pleh-oo-reh-s<u>ee</u>- yah)
pneumonia	la pulmonía (lah pool-maw-n<u>ee</u>- yah)
prescribe	recetar (reh-seh-<u>tahr</u>)
prescription	la receta (lah reh-<u>seh</u>-tah)
remain in bed	guardar cama (gwahr-<u>dahr</u> <u>kah</u>-mah)
rheumatic fever	la fiebre reumática (lah <u>fyeh</u>-breh reh-oo-<u>mah</u>-t<u>ee</u>-kah)
sample	la muestra (lah <u>mwehs</u>-trah)
shortness of breath	cortedad de aliento (kawr-teh-<u>dahd</u> deh ah-<u>lyehn</u>-taw)
(to) smoke	fumar (foo-<u>mahr</u>)
sputum	los esputos (laws ehs-<u>poo</u>-taws)
stroke	el ataque fulminante (ehl ah-<u>tah</u>- keh fool-m<u>ee</u>-<u>nahn</u>-teh)
(to) suffer	sufrir (soo-fr<u>ee</u>r)
(to) swell	hinchar (<u>ee</u>n-<u>chahr</u>)
swollen	hinchado (masculine) (<u>ee</u>n-<u>chah</u>-daw) hinchada (feminine) (<u>ee</u>n-<u>chah</u>-dah)
tea	el té (ehl teh)
(to) treat	tratar (trah-<u>tahr</u>)
treatment	el tratamiento (ehl trah-tah-<u>myehn</u>- taw)
tuberculosis	la tuberculosis (lah too-behr-koo- <u>law</u>-s<u>ee</u>s)
vomiting	los vómitos (laws <u>baw</u>-m<u>ee</u>-taws)

weak	débil (<u>deh</u>-b<u>ee</u>l)
weight	el peso (ehl <u>peh</u>-saw)
- (to lose)	perder (pehr-<u>dehr</u>)
- (to gain)	ganar (gah-<u>nahr</u>)
X-rays	los rayos equis (laws <u>rah</u>-yaws <u>eh</u>-k<u>ee</u>s)

BBB

THE DENTIST

THE DENTIST	EL DENTISTA (ehl dehn-<u>tees</u>-stah)
Sit in the chair, please!	¡Siéntese en la silla, por favor! (<u>syehn</u>-teh-seh ehn lah s<u>ee</u>-yah pawr fah-<u>bawr</u>)
What is your complaint?	¿De qué se queja? (deh keh seh <u>keh</u>-hah)
Open your mouth, please.	Abra la boca, por favor. (<u>ah</u>-brah lah <u>baw</u>-kah, pawr fah-<u>bawr</u>)
Which is the tooth that is hurting, the lower or the upper?	¿Cuál es la muela que le duele, la de abajo o la de arriba? (kwahl ehs lah <u>mweh</u>-lah keh leh <u>dweh</u>-leh, lah <u>deh</u> ah-<u>bah</u>-haw a<u>w</u> <u>lah</u> deh ahr-r<u>ee</u>-bah)
Does it hurt more when you take hot or cold things?	¿Le duele más cuando toma algo caliente o frío? (leh <u>dweh</u>-leh mahs <u>kwahn</u>-daw taw-<u>mah</u> <u>ahl</u>-gaw kahl-<u>yehn</u>-teh aw fr<u>ee</u>-aw)
Does it hurt when you chew?	¿Le duele cuando mastica? (leh <u>dweh</u>-leh <u>kwahn</u>-daw mahs-t<u>ee</u>-kah)
You have a tooth that is badly decayed.	Tiene una muela que está muy cariada. (<u>tyeh</u>-neh oo-nah <u>mweh</u>-lah keh ehs-<u>tah</u> mwy kah-r<u>ee</u>-ah-dah)
How long have you had this pain?	¿Desde cuándo tiene este dolor? (<u>dehs</u>-deh <u>kwahn</u>-daw <u>tyeh</u>-neh <u>ehs</u>-teh daw-<u>lawr</u>)
The decayed tooth will have to be extracted.	El diente cariado tiene que ser extraído. (ehl <u>dyehn</u>-teh kah-<u>ryah</u>-daw <u>tyeh</u>-neh keh <u>sehr</u> ehgs-trah-<u>ee</u>-daw)
I am going to give you an injection in the gum so that you will not feel any pain.	Le voy a dar una inyección en las encías para que no sienta ningún dolor. (leh bawy ah dahr <u>oo</u>-nah <u>een</u>-yehk-syawn ehn lahs <u>ehn</u>-s<u>ee</u>-yahs <u>pah</u>-rah keh naw <u>syehn</u>-tah n<u>ee</u>n-<u>goon</u> daw-<u>lawr</u>)
Do your gums bleed? Very much?	¿Le sangran las encías? ¿Mucho? (leh <u>sahn</u>-grahn lahs ehn-s<u>ee</u>-yahs. <u>moo</u>-chaw)
I will have to take an X-ray.	Tengo que sacar un rayo equis. (<u>tehn</u>-gaw keh sah-<u>kahr</u> oon <u>rah</u>-yaw eh-k<u>ee</u>s)

You need several fillings.	Necesita algunas empastaduras. (neh-seh-sēē-tah ahl-goo-nahs ehm-pahs-tah-doo-rahs)
I will have to use the drill.	Tengo que usar el taladro. (tehn-gaw keh oo-sahr ehl tah-lah-draw)
You need an upper (lower) denture.	Necesita una dentadura por arriba (por abajo). (neh-seh-sēē-tah oo-nah dehn-tah-doo-rah pawr ahr-rēē-bah [pawr ah-bah-haw])
You have a gum infection.	Tiene una infección de las encías. (tyeh-neh oo-nah ēēn-fehk-syawn deh lahs ehn-sēē-ahs)
I will prescribe a medicine for the infection.	Le recetaré una medicina para la infección. (leh reh-seh-tah-reh oo-nah meh-dēē-sēē-nah pah-rah lah ēēn-fehk-syawn)
You need a bridge.	Necesita un puente. (neh-seh-sēē-tah oon pwehn-teh)
Spit out!	¡Escupe! (ehs-koo-peh)
Rinse your mouth!	¡Enjuáguese la boca! (ehn-hwah-gheh-seh lah baw-kah)
I am going to clean your teeth.	Voy a limpiarle los dientes. (bawy ah lēēm-pyahr-leh laws dyehn-tehs)
Take only liquids and soft foods for 24 hours.	Tome solamente líquidos y comidas blandas por veinte y cuatro horas. (taw-meh saw-lah-mehn-teh lēē-kēē-daws y kaw-mēē-dahs blahn-dahs pawr beh-ēēn-teh ēē kwah-traw aw-rahs)
Brush your teeth after each meal.	Cepíllese los dientes después de cada comida. (seh-pēē-yeh-seh laws dyehn-tehs dehs-pwehs deh kah-dah kaw-mēē-dah)
Clean the bridge after each meal.	Límpiese el puente después de cada comida. (lēēm-pyeh-seh ehl pwehn-teh dehs-pwehs deh kah-dah kaw-mēē-dah)
I am going to give you an appointment for next week.	Voy a darle una cita para la semana próxima. (bawy ah dahr-leh oo-nah sēē-tah pah-rah lah seh-mah-nah prawk-sēē-mah)
You have pyhorrea.	Usted tiene piorrea. (oos-tehd tyeh-neh pēē-aw-reh-ah)

You will need at least five treatments.	Necesitará por lo menos cinco tratamientos. (neh-seh-see-tah-rah pawr law meh-naws seen-kaw trah-tah-myehn-taws)
I am going to give you a local anaesthetic.	Voy a darle un anestético local. (bawy ah dahr-leh oon ah-nehs-teh-tee-kaw law-kahl)
- gas	gas (gahs)
This tooth cannot be filled.	Este diente no puede ser empastado. (ehs-teh dyehn-teh naw pweh-deh sehr ehm-pahs-tah-daw)
IN THE DENTIST'S OFFICE	EN LA OFICINA DEL DENTISTA (ehn lah aw-fee-see-nah dehl dehn-tees-tah)
Useful Vocabulary	Vocabulario Útil (baw-kah-boo-lah-ryaw oo-teel)
appointment	la cita (lah see-tah)
antibiotics	los antibióticos (laws ahn-tee-byaw-tee-kaws)
bill	la cuenta (lah kwehn-tah)
(to) bleed	sangrar (sahn-grahr)
blood	la sangre (lah sahn-greh)
bridge	el puente (ehl pwehn-teh)
- removable	removible (reh-maw-bee-bleh)
- fixed	fijo (fee-haw)
(to) brush	cepillar (seh-pee-yahr)
chair	la silla (lah see-yah)
(to) chew	masticar (mahs-tee-kahr)
(to) clean	limpiar (leem-pyahr)
(to) complain	quejarse (keh-hahr-seh)
complaint	la queja (lah keh-hah)
crown	la corona (lah kaw-raw-nah)
decayed tooth	el diente cariado (ehl dyehn-teh kah-ryah-daw)
- molar	la muela cariada (lah mweh-lah kah-ryah-dah)
dental surgery	cirugía dental (see-roo-hee-ah dehn-tahl)

denture	la dentadura (lah dehn-tah-<u>doo</u>-rah)
- full	completa (kawm-<u>pleh</u>-tah)
- partial	parcial (pahr-<u>syahl</u>)
drill	el taladro (ehl tah-<u>lah</u>-draw)
(to) drill	taladrar (tah-lah-<u>drahr</u>)
(to be) extracted	ser extraído (sehr ehgs-trah-<u>ēē</u>-daw)
extraction	la extracción (lah ehgs-trahk-<u>syawn</u>)
filling	el empaste (ehl ehm-<u>pahs</u>-teh)
food	el alimento (ehl ah-<u>lēē</u>-mehn-taw)
gums	las encías (lahs ehn-<u>sēē</u>-yahs)
(to) hurt	doler (daw-<u>lehr</u>)
infection	la infección (lah <u>ēēn</u>-fehk-<u>syawn</u>)
injection	la inyección (lah <u>ēēn</u>-yehk-<u>syawn</u>)
inlay	la incrustación (lah <u>ēēn</u>-kroo-stah-<u>syawn</u>)
liquid	el líquido (ehl <u>lēē</u>-<u>kēē</u>-daw)
lower	de abajo (deh ah-<u>bah</u>-haw)
machine	el aparato (ehl ah-pah-<u>rah</u>-taw)
meal	la comida (lah kaw-<u>mēē</u>-dah)
molar	la muela (lah <u>mweh</u>-lah)
mouth	la boca (lah <u>baw</u>-kah)
- Open your mouth!	¡Abra la boca! (<u>ah</u>-brah lah <u>baw</u>-kaw)
- wider	más (mahs)
- Rinse your mouth!	¡Enjuáguese la boca! (ehn-<u>hwah</u>-gheh-seh lah <u>baw</u>-kah)
(to) need	necesitar (neh-seh-<u>sēē</u>-tahr)
pain	el dolor (ehl daw-<u>lawr</u>)
plate	la plancha (lah <u>plahn</u>-chah)
(to) prescribe	recetar (reh-seh-<u>tahr</u>)
prescription	la receta (lah reh-<u>seh</u>-tah)
pyhorrea	la piorrea (lah pyaw-<u>reh</u>-ah)

Spit out!	¡Escupa! (ehs-<u>koo</u>-pah)
soft food	comida blanda (kaw-<u>mee</u>-dah <u>blahn</u>-dah)
teeth	los dientes (laws <u>dyehn</u>-tehs)
tooth	el diente (ehl <u>dyehn</u>-teh)
toothbrush	el cepillo (ehl seh-<u>pee</u>-yaw)
treatments	los tratamientos (laws trah-tah-<u>myehn</u>-taws)
upper	de arriba (deh ah-<u>ree</u>-bah)
visit	la visita (lah b<u>ee</u>-<u>see</u>-tah)
X-rays	los rayos equis (laws <u>rah</u>-yaws <u>eh</u>-k<u>ee</u>s)

CBCB

AMBULANCE NURSE

AMBULANCE NURSE	ENFERMERA DE AMBULANCIA (ehn-fehr-<u>meh</u>-rah deh ahm-boo-<u>lahn</u>-syah)
Where is the patient?	¿Dónde está el (la) paciente? (<u>dawn</u>-deh ehs-<u>tah</u> ehl [lah] pah-<u>syehn</u>-teh)
Is the patient conscious?	¿Está consciente el (la) paciente? (ehs-tah kawn-<u>syehn</u>-teh ehl [lah] pah-<u>syehn</u>-teh)
What happened to him (her)?	¿Qué le pasó? (keh leh pah-<u>saw</u>)
When did it happen?	¿Cuándo ocurrió? (<u>kwahn</u>-daw aw-koo-<u>ryaw</u>)
How old is he (she)?	¿Qué edad tiene? (keh eh-<u>dahd</u> <u>tyeh</u>-neh)
Have you done anything for him (her)?	¿Ha hecho algo para él (ella)? (ah eh-chaw <u>ahl</u>-gaw pah-rah ehl [<u>eh</u>-yah])
Have you given him (her) any medicine?	¿Le ha dado alguna medicina? (leh ah <u>dah</u>-daw ahl-<u>goo</u>-nah meh-<u>dee</u>-<u>see</u>-nah)
Has he (she) been treated for any illness recently?	¿Ha sido tratado (tratada) para alguna enfermedad recientemente? (ah <u>see</u>-daw trah-tah-daw [trah-tah-dah] pah-rah <u>ahl</u>-goo-nah ehn-<u>fehr</u>-meh-<u>dahd</u> reh-syehn-teh-<u>mehn</u>-teh)
What is his (her) doctor's name and telephone number?	¿Cuál es el nombre y el número de teléfono de su médico? (kwahl ehs ehl <u>nawm</u>-breh <u>ee</u> ehl <u>noo</u>-meh-raw <u>deh</u> teh-leh-faw-<u>naw</u> deh soo <u>meh</u>-<u>dee</u>-kaw)
Don't move!	¡No se mueva! (naw seh <u>mweh</u>-bah)
Keep calm!	¡Cálmese! (<u>kahl</u>-meh-seh)
Everybody move away from the patient.	Todos, alárguense del (de la) paciente. (taw-daws ah-<u>lahr</u>-ghehn-seh dehl [<u>deh</u> lah] pah-<u>syehn</u>-teh)
Relax!	¡Calmese! (<u>kahl</u>-meh-seh)
We are going to put you on the stretcher.	Vamos a ponerle en la camilla. (<u>bah</u>-maws ah paw-<u>nehr</u>-leh ehn lah kah-<u>mee</u>-yah)
Can you move?	¿Puede moverse? (<u>pweh</u>-deh maw-<u>behr</u>-seh)

We will get to the hospital as
quickly as possible.

Llegaremos al hospital lo más pronto
posible. (yeh-gah-reh-maws ahl
aws-pee-tahl law mahs prawn-
taw paw-see-bleh)

Don't worry!

¡No se preocupe! (naw seh preh-
aw-koo-peh)

In the ambulance: questions
addressed to the person
accompanying the patient.

En la ambulancia: preguntas hechas
a la persona que está acompañando
al paciente. (ehn lah ahm-boo-lahn-
syah: preh-goon-tahs eh-chahs ah
lah pehr-saw-nah keh ehs-tah ah-
kawm-pahn-yahn-daw ahl pah-syehn-
teh)

What is his (her) name?

¿Cuál es su nombre? (kwahl ehs
soo nawm-breh)

What is your relationship to
the patient?

¿Cuál es el parentesco entre usted y
el (la) paciente? (kwahl ehs ehl
pah-rehn-tehs-kaw ehn-treh oos-
tehd ee ehl [lah] pah-syehn-teh)

What is the name, address and
telephone number of the
patient?

¿Cuál es el nombre, la dirección y
el número de teléfono del (de la)
paciente? (kwahl ehs ehl nawm-
breh, lah dee-rehk-syawn ee ehl
noo-meh-raw deh teh-leh-faw-
naw dehl [deh lah] pah-syehn-teh)

What is the name and telephone
number of his (her) nearest
relative or friend?

¿Cuál es el nombre y el número de
teléfono del pariente o amigo más
cercano del (de la) paciente? (kwahl
ehs ehl nawm-breh ee ehl noo-meh-
raw deh teh-leh-faw-naw dehl pah-
ryehn-teh aw ah-mee-gaw mahs
sehr-kah-naw dehl [deh lah] pah-
syehn-teh)

Does the patient have any
insurance?

¿Tiene el paciente algún seguro?
(tyeh-neh ehl pah-syehn-teh ahl-
goon seh-goo-raw)

What is the name of the insurance
company?

¿Cuál es el nombre de la compañía
de seguros? (kwahl ehs ehl nom-
breh deh lah kawm-pah-nyee-
ah deh seh-goo-raws)

What is the policy number?

¿Cuál es el número de la póliza?
(kwahl ehs ehl noo-meh-raw deh
lah paw-lee-sah)

Who will pay the expenses?

¿Quién pagará los gastos? (kyehn
pah-gah-rah laws gahs-taws)

What type of work does the
patient do?

¿Qué clase de trabajo hace el (la)
paciente? (keh klah-seh deh trah-
bah-haw ah-seh ehl [lah] pah-syehn-
teh)

What is his (her) religion?	¿ Cuál es su religión? (kwahl ehs soo reh-lee-hyawn)
Where was he (she) born?	¿ Dónde nació? (dawn-deh nah-syaw)
Is he (she) a citizen of the U.S.?	¿ Es ciudadano (ciudadana) de los Estados Unidos? (ehs syoo-dah-dah-naw syoo-dah-dah-nah deh laws ehs-tah-daws oo-nee-daws)
We have arrived at the hospital.	Hemos llegado al hospital. (eh-maws yeh-gah-daw ahl aws-pee-tahl)
They will do everything possible for you.	Harán todo lo posible para usted. (ah-rahn taw-daw law paw-see-bleh pah-rah oos-tehd)
AMBULANCE NURSE	ENFERMERA DE AMBULANCIA (ehn-fehr-meh-rah deh ahm-boo-lahn-syah)
Useful Vocabulary	Vocabulario Útil (baw-kah-boo-lah-ryaw oo-teel)
accident	el accidente (ehl ahk-see-dehn-teh)
address	la dirección (lah dee-rehk-syawn)
alive	vivo (masculine) (bee-baw) viva (feminine) (bee-bah)
ambulance	la ambulancia (lah ahm-boo-lahn-syah)
antidote	el antídoto (ehl ahn-tee-daw-taw)
(to) arrive	llegar (yeh-gahr)
artificial respiration	la respiración artificial (lah rehs-pee-rah-syawn ahr-tee-fee-syahl)
(to) assist	atender (ah-tehn-dehr)
attack	el ataque (ehl ah-tah-keh)
bandage	la venda (lah behn-dah)
(to) bandage	vendar (behn-dahr)
blanket	la manta; la frazada (lah mahn-tah; lah frah-sah-dah)
(to) bleed	sangrar (sahn-grahr)
blood	la sangre (lah sahn-greh)
broken bones	huesos rotos (weh-saws raw-taws)
Catholic	católico (masculine) (kah-taw-lee-kaw) católica (feminine) (kah-taw-lee-kah)

citizen of the United States	ciudadano de los Estados Unidos (syoo-dah-dah-naw deh laws ehs-tah-daws oo-nee-daws) ciudadana (feminine) (syoo-dah-dah-nah)
convulsion	el espasmo (ehl ehs-pahs-maw)
dead	muerto (masculine) (mwehr-taw) muerta (feminine) (mwehr-tah)
doctor	el médico (ehl meh-dee-kaw)
drugs	las drogas (lahs draw-gahs)
expenses	los gastos (laws gahs-taws)
(to) faint	desmayarse (dehs-mah-yahr-seh)
first aid	los primeros auxilios (laws pree-meh-raws ah-oo-see-lyaws)
friend	el amigo (masculine) (ehl ah-mee-gaw) la amiga (feminine) (lah ah-mee-gah)
(to) happen	ocurrir; pasar (aw-koo-reer. pah-sahr)
help	la ayuda (lah ah-yoo-dah)
hospital	el hospital (ehl aws-pee-tahl)
(to) hurt	doler (daw-lehr)
illness	la enfermedad (lah ehn-fehr-meh-dahd)
insurance company	la compañía de seguros (lah kawm-pan-yee-ah deh seh-goo-raws)
murder	el asesinato (ehl ah-seh-see-nah-taw)
(to) move	moverse (maw-behr-seh)
name	el nombre (ehl nawm-breh)
pain	el dolor (ehl daw-lawr)
(to) pay	pagar (pah-gahr)
patient	el (la) paciente (ehl [lah] pah-syehn-teh)
priest	el cura; el sacerdote (ehl koo-rah; ehl sah-sehr-daw-teh)
Protestant	protestante (praw-tehs-tahn-teh)

Quiet!	¡Silencio! (see-lehn-syaw)
relationship	el parentesco (ehl pah-rehn-tehs-kaw)
relative	el (la) pariente (ehl [lah] pah-ryehn-teh)
religion	la religión (lah reh-lee-hyawn)
(to) save	salvar (sahl-bahr)
stretcher	la camilla (lah kah-mee-yah)
suddenly	de repente (deh reh-pehn-teh)
suicide	el suicidio (ehl sooy-see-dyaw)
symptoms	los síntomas (laws seen-taw-mahs)
telephone	el teléfono (ehl teh-leh-faw-naw)
time	el tiempo (ehl tyehm-paw)
tourniquet	el torniquete (ehl tawr-nee-keh-teh)
unconscious	inconsciente (een-kawn-syehn-teh)
work	el empleo; el trabajo (ehl ehm-pleh-aw; ehl trah-bah-haw)
(to) work	trabajar (trah-bah-hahr)
wound	la herida (lah eh-ree-dah)
wounded	herido (masculine) (eh-ree-daw) herida (feminine) (eh-ree-dah)

BBB

THE DIETICIAN

THE DIETICIAN	LA CONSEJERA DE ALIMENTOS (lah kawn-seh-heh-rah deh ah-lee-mehn-taws)
Good morning! How do you feel today?	¿Buenos días! Cómo se siente hoy? (bweh-naws dee-ahs. kaw-maw seh syehn-teh awy)
Are you happy with your food?	¿ Está contento (contenta) con la comida? (ehs-tah kawn-tehn-taw [kawn-tehn-tah] kawn lah kaw-mee-dah)
Are you served enough?	¿ Le sirven bastante? (leh seer-behn bahs-tahn-teh)
Would you like something else between meals?	¿Quisiera algo más entre comidas? (kee-syeh-rah ahl-gaw mahs ehn-treh kaw-mee-dahs)
- Milk?	¿Leche? (leh-cheh)
- Orange juice?	¿Jugo de naranja? (hoo-gaw deh nah-rahn-hah)
- Apple juice?	¿Jugo de manzana? (hoo-gaw deh mahn-sah-nah)
- Pineapple juice?	¿Jugo de piña? (hoo-gaw deh pee-nyah)
- Grapefruit juice?	¿Jugo de toronja? (hoo-gaw deh taw-rawn-hah)
- Jell-o?	¿Gelatina? (heh-lah-tee-nah)
- Custard?	¿Flan? (flahn)
What quantity of liquids do you take daily?	¿Qué cantidad de líquidos toma usted por día? (keh kahn-tee-dahd deh lee-kee-daws taw-mah oos-tehd pawr dee-yah)
What type of liquids do you take?	¿Qué clase de líquidos toma? (keh klah-seh deh lee-kee-daws taw-mah)
- Water?	¿ Agua? (ah-gwah)
- Milk?	¿ Leche? (leh-cheh)
- Fruit juices?	¿ Jugo de frutas? (hoo-gaw deh froo-tahs)
- Coffee?	¿ Café? (kah-feh)
- Tea?	¿ Té? (teh)

Is there any food that we serve you that upsets your stomach?

¿Hay algo en la comida que le servimos que le moleste el estómago? (ahy ahl-gaw ehn lah kaw-_mee_-dah keh leh sehr-_bee_-maws keh leh maw-_lehs_-teh ehl ehs-_taw_-mah-gaw)

The meals that you are served conform to your doctor's specifications.

Las comidas que le sirven aquí están de acuerdo con las especificaciones de su médico. (lahs kaw-_mee_-dahs keh leh _seer_-behn ah-_kee_ ehs-_tahn_ deh ah-_kwehr_-daw kawn lahs ehs-peh-_see-fee-kah-syaw_-nehs deh soo meh-_dee_-kaw)

If you wish any changes in your diet, please consult your doctor.

Si quisiera algún cambio en su régimen, por favor consulte a su médico. (see _kee_-syeh-rah ahl-_goon_ kahm-byaw ehn soo reh-_hee_-mehn pawr fah-bawr kawn-_sool_-teh ah soo meh-_dee_-kaw)

THE DIETICIAN

LA CONSEJERA DE ALIMENTOS (lah kawn-seh-_heh_-rah deh ah-_lee_-mehn-taws)

Useful Vocabulary

Vocabulario Útil (baw-kah-boo-_lah_-ryaw oo-_teel_)

apple

la manzana (lah mahn-_sah_-nah)

bacon

el tocino (ehl taw-_see_-naw)

beef

la carne de vaca (lah _kahr_-neh deh _bah_-kah)

beets

las remolachas (lahs reh-maw-_lah_-chahs)

bread

el pan (ehl pahn)

breakfast

el desayuno (ehl deh-sah-_yoo_-naw)

butter

la mantequilla (lah mahn-teh-_kee_-yah)

cabbage

la col (lah kawl)

calorie

la caloría (lah kah-law-_ree_-ah)

carbohydrate

carbohidrato (kahr-baw-_ee_-drah-taw)

carrots

las zanahorias (lahs sah-nah-_aw_-ryahs)

cauliflower

la coliflor (lah kaw-_lee_-flawr)

celery

el apio (ehl _ah_-pyaw)

cereal

el cereal (ehl seh-reh-_ahl_)

cheese	el queso (ehl <u>keh</u>-saw)
chicken	el pollo (ehl <u>paw</u>-yaw)
chicken soup	el caldo de gallina (ehl <u>kahl</u>-daw deh gah-<u>yee</u>-nah)
cholesterol	el colesterol (ehl kaw-lehs-teh-<u>rawl</u>)
chops	las costillas (lahs kaw-<u>stee</u>-yahs)
coffee	el café (ehl kah-<u>feh</u>)
daily	por día; cada día (pawr <u>dee</u>-yah; kah-dah <u>dee</u>-yah)
diabetes	la diabetes (lah <u>dee</u>-ah-<u>beh</u>-tehs)
dessert	el postre (ehl <u>paw</u>-streh)
diet	el régimen; la dieta (ehl <u>reh</u>-hee-mehn; la <u>dyeh</u>-tah)
(to be on a) diet	estar a dieta (ehs-<u>tahr</u> ah <u>dyeh</u>-tah)
dinner	la cena (lah <u>seh</u>-nah)
eggs	los huevos (laws <u>weh</u>-baws)
- fried	fritos (<u>free</u>-taws)
- hard boiled	duros (<u>doo</u>-raws)
- omelette	tortilla (tawr-<u>tee</u>-yah)
- poached	escalfados (ehs-kahl-<u>fah</u>-daws)
- scrambled	revueltos (reh-<u>bwehl</u>-taws)
- soft boiled	pasados por agua (pah-sah-daws pawr <u>ah</u>-gwah)
fat	gordo (masculine) (<u>gawr</u>-daw) gorda (feminine) (<u>gawr</u>-dah)
fish	el pescado (ehl pehs-<u>kah</u>-daw)
food	el alimento (ehl ah-<u>lee</u>-<u>mehn</u>-taw)
food poisoning	intoxicación por comestibles (<u>een</u>-tawk-<u>see</u>-kah-<u>syawn</u> pawr kaw-mehs-<u>tee</u>-blehs)
gastric ulcer	la úlcera gástrica (lah <u>ool</u>-seh-rah <u>gahs</u>-<u>tree</u>-kah)
ham	el jamón (ehl hah-<u>mawn</u>)
heartburn	el ardor del estómago (ehl ahr-<u>dawr</u> dehl ehs-<u>taw</u>-mah-gaw)

(to be) hungry	tener hambre (teh-<u>nehr</u> ahm-breh)
ice cream	el helado (ehl eh-<u>lah</u>-daw)
iced water	agua con hielo (<u>ah</u>-gwah kawn <u>yeh</u>-law)
indigestion	la indigestión (lah een-dee-hehs- tyawn)
lamb	carne de cordero (<u>kahr</u>-neh deh kawr-deh-raw)
lettuce	la lechuga (lah leh-<u>choo</u>-gah)
liquids	los líquidos (laws lee-kee-daws)
lunch	el almuerzo (ehl ahl-<u>mwehr</u>-saw)
(to have) lunch	tomar el almuerzo (taw-<u>mahr</u> ehl ahl-mwehr-saw)
malnutrition	la desnutrición (lah dehs-noo-tree- syawn)
meal	la comida (lah kaw-mee-dah)
meat	la carne (lah <u>kahr</u>-neh)
milk	la leche (lah <u>leh</u>-cheh)
minerals	los minerales (laws mee-neh-<u>rah</u>- lehs)
peaches	los melocotones (laws meh-law-kaw- <u>taw</u>-nehs)
pears	las peras (lahs <u>peh</u>-rahs)
peas	los guisantes (laws ghee-<u>sahn</u>-tehs)
pork	carne de cerdo (<u>kahr</u>-neh deh <u>sehr</u>- daw)
potatoes	las papas (lahs <u>pah</u>-pahs)
proteins	las proteínas (lahs praw-teh-ee- nahs)
quantity	la cantidad (lah kahn-tee-<u>dahd</u>)
rice	el arroz (ehl ahr-<u>raws</u>)
salad	la ensalada (lah ehn-sah-<u>lah</u>-dah)
salt	la sal (lah sahl)
(to be) satisfied	estar satisfecho (a) (ehs-<u>tahr</u> sah- tees-<u>feh</u>-chaw [ah])
soup	el caldo (ehl <u>kahl</u>-daw)

spinach	las espinacas (lahs ehs-pēē-nah-kahs)
steak	el biftec; bistec (ehl bēēf-tehk; bēēs-tehk)
stomach	el estómago (ehl ehs-taw-mah-gaw)
string beans	las habichuelas (lahs ah-bēē-chweh-lahs)
tea	el té (ehl teh)
thin	delgado; flaco (masculine) (dehl-gah-daw; flah-kaw) delgada; flaca (feminine) (dehl-gah-dah; flah-kah)
(to be) thirsty	tener sed (teh-nehr sehd)
toast	el pan tostado (ehl pahn taw-stah-daw)
tomato	el tomate (ehl taw-mah-teh)
too much	demasiado (deh mah-syah-daw)
turkey	el pavo (ehl pah-baw)
veal	carne de ternera (kahr-neh deh tehr-neh-rah)
- cutlets	chuletas de ternera (choo-leh-tahs deh tehr-neh-rah)
vegetables	las legumbres (lahs leh-goom-brehs)
vegetarian	vegetariano (beh-heh-tah-ryah-naw)
vitamins	las vitaminas (lahs bēē-tah-mēē-nahs)
water	el agua (ehl ah-gwah)
- cold	fría (frēē-ah)
- hot	caliente (kah-lyehn-teh)
(to gain) weight	ganar peso (gah-nahr peh-saw)
(to lose) weight	perder peso (pehr-dehr peh-saw)

THE PHYSICAL THERAPIST

PHYSICAL THERAPY	LA TERAPIA FÍSICA (lah teh-rah-pyah fee-see-kah)
What is your name?	¿Cómo se llama? (kaw-maw seh yah-mah)
How old are you?	¿Cuántos años tiene? (kwahn-taws ahn-yaws tyeh-neh)
What is your problem?	¿Cuál es su problema? (kwahl ehs soo praw-bleh-mah)
I am going to try to help you.	Voy a tratar de ayudarle. (bawy ah trah-tahr deh ah-yoo-dahr-leh)
We shall do the exercises gradually.	Vamos a hacer los ejercicios poco a poco. (bah-maws ah ah-sehr laws eh-hehr-see-syaws paw-kaw ah paw-kaw)
Relax!	¡Relájese! (reh-lah-heh-seh)
This won't hurt you.	Esto no le va a doler. (ehs-taw naw leh bah ah daw-lehr)
This will hurt a little.	Esto le va a doler un poquito. (ehs-taw leh bah ah daw-lehr oon paw-kee-taw)
Do you feel anything?	¿Siente algo? (syehn-teh ahl-gaw)
Do you feel any pain?	¿Siente algún dolor? (syehn-teh ahl-goon daw-lawr)
Good!	¡Bueno! (bweh-naw)
Now let's work together!	¡Ahora vamos a trabajar juntos! (ah-aw-rah bah-maws ah trah-bah-hahr hoon-taws)
First, move the big toe.	Primero, mueva usted el dedo grueso del pie. (pree-meh-raw mweh-bah oos-tehd ehl deh-daw grweh-saw dehl pyeh)
- the toes	los dedos del pie (laws deh-daws dehl pyeh)
- the foot	el pie (ehl pyeh)
- the feet	los pies (laws pyehs)
- the leg	la pierna (lah pyehr-nah)
- the legs	las piernas (lahs pyehr-nahs)
- the finger	el dedo (ehl deh-daw)
- the fingers	los dedos (laws deh-daws)

- the hand	la mano (lah mah-naw)
- the hands	las manos (lahs mah-naws)
- the head	la cabeza (lah kah-beh-sah)
- the hip	la cadera (lah kah-deh-rah)
- the shoulder	el hombro (ehl awm-braw)
- right	derecho (derecha) (deh-reh-chaw [deh-reh-chah])
- left	izquierdo (izquierda) (ees-kyehr-daw [ees-kyehr-dah])
- to the right	a la derecha (ah lah deh-reh-chah)
- to the left	a la izquierda (ah lah ees-kyehr-dah)
Good effort!	¡Buen esfuerzo! (bwehn ehs-fwehr-saw)
Please try a little harder!	¡Por favor, haga un poco más esfuerzo! (pawr fah-bawr hah-gah oon paw-kaw mahs ehs-fwehr-saw)
Let's try the exercise now.	Vamos a hacer el ejercicio ahora. (bah-maws ah ah-sehr ehl eh-hehr-see-syaw ah-aw-rah)
Please watch how I do it!	¡Mire como lo hago yo! (mee-reh kaw-maw law hah-gaw yaw)
Shall I do it once more?	¿Lo hago otra vez? (law hah-gaw aw-trah vehs)
Watch carefully!	¡Fíjese! (fee-heh-seh)
Now you do it!	¡Ahora hágalo usted! (ah-aw-rah ah-gah-law oos-tehd)
Very good!	¡Muy bien! (mwee byehn)
Rest!	¡Descanse! (dehs-kahn-seh)
Sit down!	¡Siéntese! (syehn-teh-seh)
Stand up!	¡Levántese! (leh-bahn-teh-seh)
Remain standing!	¡Quédese de pie! (keh-deh-seh deh pyeh)
Walk!	¡Camine usted! (kah-mee-neh oos-tehd)
Stand on tiptoe!	¡Póngase en puntillas! (pawn-gah-seh ehn poon-tee-yahs)

Lie down!	¡Acuéstese! (ah-<u>kwehs</u>-teh-seh)
Turn over on your stomach!	¡Voltéese boca abajo! (bawl-<u>teh</u>-eh-seh <u>baw</u>-kah ah-<u>bah</u>-haw)
Turn over on your back!	¡Voltéese boca arriba! (bawl-<u>teh</u>-eh-seh <u>baw</u>-kah ah-<u>ree</u>-bah)
Lift up your head!	¡Levante la cabeza! (leh-<u>bahn</u>-teh lah kah-<u>beh</u>-sah)
- your arm	el brazo (ehl <u>brah</u>-saw)
- your leg	la pierna (lah <u>pyehr</u>-nah)
- your buttocks	las nalgas (lahs <u>nahl</u>-gahs)
Push!	¡Empuje! (ehm-<u>poo</u>-heh)
Pull!	¡Tire! (<u>tee</u>-reh)
Stretch!	¡Estírese usted! (ehs-<u>tee</u>-reh-seh oos-<u>tehd</u>)
Kick!	¡Patée! (pah-teh-eh)
Jump!	¡Salte! (<u>sahl</u>-teh)
Excellent! You are making progress!	¡Excelente! Está haciendo progresos! (ehk-seh-<u>lehn</u>-teh. ehs-<u>tah</u> ah-<u>syehn</u>-daw praw-<u>greh</u>-saws)
Bend your wrist!	¡Doble la muñeca! (<u>daw</u>-bleh lah moon-<u>yeh</u>-kah)
- your elbow	el codo (ehl <u>kaw</u>-daw)
- your knee	la rodilla (lah raw-<u>dee</u>-yah)
More, please!	¡Más, por favor! (mahs pawr fah-<u>bawr</u>)
Move over to the machine!	¡Acérquese usted a la máquina! (ah-<u>sehr</u>-keh-seh oos-<u>tehd</u> ah lah <u>mah</u>-<u>kee</u>-nah)
Go into the water slowly!	¡Entre en el agua despacio! (<u>ehn</u>-treh ehn ehl ah-gwah dehs-<u>pah</u>-syaw)
Do you need help?	¿Necesita ayuda? (neh-seh-<u>see</u>-tah ah-<u>yoo</u>-dah)
Are you comfortable?	¿Está cómodo (cómoda)? (ehs-tah <u>kaw</u>-maw-daw [<u>kaw</u>-maw-dah])
Why not?	¿Por qué no? (pawr keh naw)
Until tomorrow!	¡Hasta mañana! (<u>ahs</u>-tah mahn-<u>yah</u>-nah)

It's been a pleasure helping you.

Ha sido un gran placer ayudarle.
(ah <u>see</u>-daw oon grahn plah-<u>sehr</u>
ah-yoo-<u>dahr</u>-leh)

Goodbye!

¡Adios! (ah-<u>dyaws</u>)

PHYSICAL THERAPY

LA TERAPIA FISICA
(lah teh-<u>rah</u>-pyah <u>fee</u>-<u>see</u>-kah)

Useful Vocabulary

Vocabulario Útil
(baw-kah-boo-<u>lah</u>-ryaw <u>oo</u>-<u>tee</u>l)

age

la edad (lah eh-<u>dahd</u>)

(to) bend

doblar (daw-<u>blahr</u>)

Be careful!

¡Cuidado! (kw<u>ee</u>-<u>dah</u>-daw)

disability

la incapacidad (lah <u>ee</u>n-kah-pah-
<u>see</u>-<u>dahd</u>)

effort

el esfuerzo (ehl ehs-<u>fwehr</u>-saw)

(to make) an effort

hacer un esfuerzo (ah-<u>sehr</u> oon
ehs-<u>fwehr</u>-saw)

(to) feel

sentir (sehn-<u>tee</u>r)

feeling

la sensación (lah sehn-sah-<u>syawn</u>)

gradually

poco a poco (<u>paw</u>-kaw ah <u>paw</u>-kaw)

(to) help

ayudar (ah-yoo-<u>dahr</u>)

injury

la lesión (lah leh-<u>syawn</u>)

(to) jump

saltar (sahl-<u>tahr</u>)

left

izquierdo [izquierda] (<u>ee</u>s-<u>kyehr</u>-daw
[<u>ee</u>s-<u>kyehr</u>-dah])

(to) move

mover (maw-<u>behr</u>)

(to) need

necesitar (neh-seh-<u>see</u>-<u>tahr</u>)

numbness

el adormecimiento (ehl ah-dawr-
meh-see-<u>myehn</u>-taw)

pain

el dolor (ehl daw-<u>lawr</u>)

problem

el problema (ehl praw-<u>bleh</u>-mah)

(to) pull

tirar (t<u>ee</u>-<u>rahr</u>)

(to) push

empujar (ehm-poo-<u>hahr</u>)

quickly

rápidamente (<u>rah</u>-p<u>ee</u>-dah-mehn-
teh)

relax

relajar (reh-lah-<u>hahr</u>)

(to) rest	descansar (dehs-kahn-<u>sahr</u>)
slowly	despacio (dehs-<u>pah</u>-syaw)
(to) stretch	estirar (ehs-tee-<u>rahr</u>)
(to) touch	tocar (taw-<u>kahr</u>)
(to) try	tratar de (trah-<u>tahr</u> deh)
(to) watch carefully	fijarse (fee-<u>hahr</u>-seh)

CBB

THE RECEPTIONIST AT INFORMATION DESK

THE RECEPTIONIST	LA RECEPCIONISTA
	(lah reh-sehp-syaw-nēēs-tah)

Good morning! — ¡Buenos días! (bweh-naws dēē-ahs)

Good afternoon! — ¡Buenas tardes! (bweh-nahs tahr-dehs)

Good evening! — ¡Buenas noches! (bweh-nahs naw-chehs)

May I help you? — ¿En qué puedo servirle? (ehn keh pweh-daw sehr-bēēr-leh)

Mr. --- (Mrs. ---; Miss ---) is in Room ---; on the first (second, third, fourth) floor. — El señor --- (la señora ---; la señorita ---) está en cuarto número ---; en el primer (segundo, tercer cuarto) piso. (ehl sehn-yawr [lah sehn-yaw-rah; lah sehn-yawr-rēē-tah] ehs-tah ehn kwahr-taw noo-meh-raw; ehn ehl prēē-mehr [seh-goon-daw, tehr-sehr, kwahr-taw] pēē-saw)

The patient is under intensive care. — El (la) paciente está bajo cuidado intensivo. (ehl [lah] pah-syehn-teh ehs-tah bah-haw kwēē-dah-daw ēēn-tehn-sēē-baw)

No visitors are allowed except the immediate family. — No puede recibir visitas fuera de los miembros más cercanos de la familia. (naw pweh-deh reh-sēē-bēēr bēē-sēē-tahs fweh-rah deh laws myehm-braws mahs sehr-kah-naws deh lah fah-mēēl-yah)

The patient was discharged this morning. — El (la) paciente fue despedido (despedida) esta mañana. (ehl [lah] pah-syehn-teh fweh dehs-peh-dēē-daw [dehs-peh-dēē-dah] ehs-tah mahn-yah-nah)

You must obtain a pass before visiting the patient. — Usted tiene que obtener un pase antes de visitar al (a la) paciente. (oos-tehd tyeh-neh keh awb-teh-nehr oon pah-seh ahn-tehs deh bēē-sēē-tahr ahl [ah lah] pah-syehn-teh)

The patient may not have more than two (three) visitors at a time. — El (la) paciente no puede recibir más de dos (tres) visitas a la vez. (ehl [lah] pah-syehn-teh naw pweh-deh reh-sēē-bēēr mahs deh daws [trehs] bēē-sēē-tahs ah lah behs)

The visiting hours are from _____ to _____ in the afternoon; and from _____ to _____ in the evening.

Las horas de visita son desde las _____ hasta las _____ de la tarde; y desde las _____ y las _____ de la noche. (lahs aw-rahs deh bee-see-tah sawn dehz-deh lahs _____ ahs-tah lahs _____ deh lah tahr-deh; ee dehz-deh lahs _____ ee lahs _____ deh lah naw-cheh)

When the bell rings you must leave.

Cuando suena el timbre tiene que salir. (kwahn-daw sweh-nah ehl teem-breh tyeh-neh keh sah-leer)

Children are not allowed to visit the patient.

No se permite que los niños visiten al paciente. (naw seh pehr-mee-teh keh laws neen-yaws bee-see-tehn ahl pah-syen-teh)

There is a waiting room on the first (second, third) floor.

Hay una sala de espera en el primer (segundo, tercer) piso. (ahy oo-nah sah-lah deh ehs-peh-rah ehn ehl pree-mehr [seh-goon-daw, tehr-sehr] pee-saw)

There is a gift shop on the first floor.

Hay una tienda de regalos en el primer piso. (ahy oo-nah tyehn-dah deh reh-gah-laws ehn ehl pree-mehr pee-saw

It is open from _____ to _____ every day.

Está abierta desde las _____ hasta las _____ cada día. (ehs-tah ah-byehr-tah dehz-deh lahs _____ ahs-tah lahs _____ kah-dah dee-ah)

The cafeteria is on the ground floor.

La cafetería está en el piso bajo. (lah kah-feh-teh-ree-ah ehs-tah ehn ehl pee-saw bah-haw)

The elevator to all floors is to the left.

El ascensor que va a todos los pisos está a la izquierda. (ehl ah-sehn-sawr keh bah ah taw-daws laws pee-saws ehs-tah ah lah ees-kyehr-dah)

- to the right

a la derecha (ah lah deh-reh-chah)

- straight ahead

derecho (deh-reh-chaw)

The chapel is on the ground floor.

La capilla está en el piso bajo. (lah kah-pee-yah ehs-tah ehn ehl pee-saw bah-haw)

The patient's telephone number is _____

El número de teléfono del (de la) paciente es _____ (ehl noo-meh-raw deh teh-leh-faw-naw dehl [deh lah] pah-syehn-teh ehs_____)

I shall call Dr. _____ over the loudspeaker.	Llamaré al doctor _____ por el altoparlante. (yah-mah-reh ahl dawk-tawr _____ pawr ehl ahl-taw-pahr-lahn-teh)
Here are the passes.	Aquí están los pases. (ah-kee ehs-tahn laws pah-sehs)
You're welcome.	De nada. (deh nah-dah)
THE RECEPTIONIST	LA RECEPCIONISTA (lah reh-sehp-syaw-nees-tah)
Useful Vocabulary	Vocabulario Útil (baw-kah-boo-lah-ryaw oo-teel)
(to) assist	ayudar (ah-yoo-dahr)
bathroom	el cuarto de baño (ehl kwahr-taw deh bahn-yaw)
bell	el timbre (ehl teem-breh)
cafeteria	la cafetería (lah kah-feh-teh-ree-ah)
(to) call	llamar (yah-mahr)
chapel	la capilla (lah kah-pee-yah)
children	los niños (laws neen-yaws)
condition	la condición (lah kawn-dee-syawn)
doctor	el médico (ehl meh-dee-kaw)
door	la puerta (lah pwehr-tah)
elevator	el ascensor (ehl ah-sehn-sawr)
extension	la extensión (lah ehgs-tehn-syawn)
floor	el piso (ehl pee-saw)
- first	el primer piso (ehl pree-mehr pee-saw)
- second	el segundo (ehl seh-goon-daw)
- third	el tercer (ehl tehr-sehr)
- fourth	el cuarto (ehl kwahr-taw)
- fifth	el quinto (ehl keen-taw)
friend	el amigo (masculine) (ehl ah-mee-gaw)
	la amiga (feminine) (lah ah-mee-gah)

gift shop	la tienda de regalos (lah tyehn-dah deh reh-gah-laws)
guard	el guardia (ehl gwahr-dyah)
(to) help	ayudar (ah-yoo-dahr)
hour	la hora (lah aw-rah)
immediate family	los miembros más cercano de la familia. (laws myehm-braws mahs sehr-kah-naws deh lah fah-meel-yah)
information	la información (lah een-fawr-mah-syawn)
intensive care	el cuidado intensivo. (ehl kwee-dah-daw een-tehn-see-baw)
(to) leave	salir (sah-leer)
left (to the)	a la izquierda (ah lah ees-kyehr-dah)
loudspeaker	el altoparlante (ehl ahl-taw-pahr-lahn-teh)
man	el hombre (ehl awm-breh)
name	el nombre (ehl nawm-breh)
number	el número (ehl noo-meh-raw)
nurse	la enfermera (lah ehn-fehr-meh-rah)
(to) obtain	obtener (awb-teh-nehr)
pass	el pase (ehl pah-seh)
patient	el (la) paciente (ehl [lah] pah-syehn-teh)
permitted (it is not)	no se permite. (naw seh pehr-mee-teh)
relative	el (la) pariente (ehl [lah] pah-ryehn-teh)
right (to the)	a la derecha (ah lah deh-reh-chah)
room	el cuarto (ehl kwahr-taw)
silence	silencio (see-lehn-syaw)
straight ahead	derecho (deh-reh-chaw)
stairway	la escalera (lah ehs-kah-leh-rah)

telephone number   el número de teléfono (ehl noo-meh-raw deh teh-leh-faw-naw)

(to) wait   esperar (ehs-peh-rahr)

waiting room   la sala de espera (lah sah-lah deh ehs-peh-rah)

(to) visit   visitar (bee-see-tahr)

visiting hours   las horas de visita (lahs aw-rahs deh bee-see-tah)

woman   la mujer (lah moo-hehr)

ⅬⅬⅬ

WORKMEN'S COMPENSATION

WORKMEN'S COMPENSATION

Report of Injury	Información sobre el accidente (ēēn-fawr-mah-syawn saw-breh ehl ahk-sēē-dehn-teh)
Last name?	¿El apellido? (ehl ah-peh-yēē-daw)
First name?	¿Nombre? (nawm-breh)
Address?	¿Domicilio? (daw-mēē-sēē-lyaw)
Social Security number?	¿El número del sequro social? (ehl noo-meh-raw dehl seh-goo-raw saw-syahl)
Age?	¿Edad? (eh-dahd)
Employer?	¿El jefe? (ehl heh-feh)
- The company?	¿La compañía? (lah kawm-pahn-yēē-ah)
- Address?	¿La dirección? (lah dēē-rehk-syawn)
- Telephone number?	¿El número de teléfono? (ehl noo-meh-raw deh teh-leh-faw-naw)
Your occupation?	¿Su oficio? (soo aw-fēē-syaw)
Insurance carrier?	¿El nombre de la compañía de seguros? (ehl nawm-breh deh lah kawm-pahn-yee-ah deh seh-goo-raws)
Where did the accident occur?	¿Dónde ocurrió el accidente? (dawn-deh aw-koo-ryaw ehl ahk-sēē-dehn-teh)
Date?	¿La fecha? (lah feh-chah)
Day of the week?	¿El día de la semana? (ehl dēē-ah deh lah seh-mah-nah)
The hour?	¿La hora? (lah aw-rah)
- A.M.?	¿De la mañana? (deh lah man-yah-nah)
- P.M.?	¿De la noche? (deh lah naw-cheh)
When did your disability begin?	¿Cuándo empezó su incapacidad? (kwahn-daw ehm-peh-saw soo ēēn-kah-pah-sēē-dahd)
Did they pay you for the whole day?	¿Le han pagado por el día entero del accidente? (leh ahn pah-gah-daw pawr ehl dēē-ah ehn-teh-raw dehl ahk-sēē-dehn-teh)

Please describe the accident.

Por favor, describa usted el accidente.
(pawr fah-bawr dehs-kree-bah oos-tehd ehl ahk-see-dehn-teh)

What were you doing when the accident occurred?

¿Qué hacía usted cuando ocurrió el accidente? (keh ah-see-ah oos-tehd kwahn-daw aw-koo-ryaw ehl ahk-see-dehn-teh)

What machine or object caused the accident?

¿Qué máquina o objeto causó el accidente? (keh mah-kee-nah aw awb-heh-taw kah-oo-saw ehl ahk-see-dehn-teh)

ℰℬℬ

COMMANDS

COMMANDS	MANDOS (mahn-daws)
Let me see!	¡Déjeme ver! (deh-heh-meh behr)
Show me where it hurts!	¡Enséñeme donde le duele! (ehn-sehn-yeh-meh dawn-deh leh dweh-leh)
Listen!	¡Oiga! (awy-gah)
Speak slowly, please!	¡Hable despacio, por favor! (ah-bleh dehs-pah-syaw pawr fah-bawr)
Answer only "yes" or "no"!	¡Conteste solamente "sí" o "no"! (kawn-tehs-teh saw-lah-mehn-teh see aw naw)
Say "ah"!	¡Diga "ah"! (dēē-gah ah)
Take a deep breath!	¡Respire profundamente! (rehs-pēē-reh praw-foon-dah-mehn-teh)
Hold your breath!	¡No respire! (naw rehs-pēē-reh)
Please breathe normally!	Por favor, ¡respire normalmente! (pawr fah-bawr rehs-pēē-reh nawr-mahl-mehn-teh)
Open your mouth!	¡Abra la boca! (ah-brah lah baw-kah)
Cough!	¡Tosa! (taw-sah)
Sit down!	¡Siéntese! (syehn-teh-seh)
Stand up!	¡Levántese! (leh-bahn-teh-seh)
Walk a little!	¡Camine un poco! (kah-mēē-neh oon paw-kaw)
Take this!	¡Tome éste! (taw-meh ehs-teh)
Raise your arm!	¡Levante el brazo! (leh-bahn-teh ehl brah-saw) ·
Don't worry!	¡No se preocupe! (naw seh preh-aw-koo-peh)
Bathe in warm (cold) water!	¡Báñese en agua tibia (fría)! (bahn-yeh-seh ehn ah-gwah tēē-byah [frēē-ah])
Close your hand!	¡Cierre la mano! (syeh-reh lah mah-naw)
Make a fist!	¡Haga un puño! (ah-gah oon poon-yaw)

Open it!	¡Ábrala! (<u>ah</u>-brah-lah)
Lie down!	¡Acuéstese! (ah-<u>kwehs</u>-teh-seh)
Lie on your left side!	¡Acuéstese sobre el lado izquierdo! (ah-<u>kwehs</u>-<u>t</u>eh-seh saw-breh ehl <u>lah</u>-daw <u>ees</u>-<u>kyehr</u>-daw)
- right side	el lado derecho (ehl <u>lah</u>-daw deh-<u>reh</u>-chaw)
Turn over!	¡Vírese del otro lado! (b<u>ee</u>-reh-seh dehl <u>aw</u>-traw <u>lah</u>-daw)
Stretch your legs!	¡Estire las piernas! (ehs-t<u>ee</u>-reh lahs <u>pyehr</u>-nahs)
Bend your head to the right!	¡Doble la cabeza a la derecha! (daw-bleh lah kah-<u>beh</u>-sah ah lah deh-<u>reh</u>-chah)
- to the left	a la izquierda (ah lah <u>ees</u>-<u>kyehr</u>-dah)
- forward	hacia adelante (<u>ah</u>-syah ah-deh-<u>lahn</u>-teh)
- backward	hacia atras (<u>ah</u>-syah ah-<u>trahs</u>)
Exercise like this!	¡Haga ejercicios así! (<u>ah</u>-gah eh-hehr-<u>see</u>-syaws ah-s<u>ee</u>)
Turn over!	¡Vírese del otro lado! (b<u>ee</u>-reh-seh dehl <u>aw</u>-traw <u>lah</u>-daw)
Sign here, please!	¡Firme aquí, por favor! (f<u>ee</u>r-meh ah-k<u>ee</u> pawr fah-<u>bawr</u>)
Wait a moment!	¡Espere un momento! (ehs-<u>peh</u>-reh oon maw-<u>mehn</u>-taw)
Please fill out these forms.	Favor de llenar estas planillas. (fah-<u>bawr</u> deh yeh-<u>nahr</u> <u>ehs</u>-tahs plah-<u>nee</u>-yahs)
Remove your clothes!	¡Quítese la ropa! (k<u>ee</u>-teh-seh lah <u>raw</u>-pah)
Put on the gown!	¡Póngase el camisón! (<u>pawn</u>-gah-seh ehl kah-m<u>ee</u>-<u>sawn</u>)
Do not climb stairs!	¡No suba escaleras! (naw <u>soo</u>-bah ehs-kah-<u>leh</u>-rahs)
Explain how it happened!	¡Explíqueme cómo ocurrió! (ehgs-<u>plee</u>-keh-meh <u>kaw</u>-maw aw-koo-<u>ryaw</u>)
Bend over!	¡Dóblese! (<u>daw</u>-bleh-seh)
Bend your knees!	¡Doble las rodillas! (<u>daw</u>-bleh lahs raw-d<u>ee</u>-yahs)

Bend your elbows!	¡Doble los codos! (daw-bleh laws <u>kaw</u>-daws)
Stay in bed!	¡Quédese en cama! (<u>keh</u>-deh-seh ehn <u>kah</u>-mah)
Come in!	¡Entre usted! (<u>ehn</u>-treh oos-tehd)
Don't eat sugar or sweets!	¡No coma ni azúcar ni dulces! (naw <u>kaw</u>-mah nē̄ē ah-<u>soo</u>-kahr nē̄ē <u>dool</u>-sehs)
Get down from the table!	¡Bájese de la mesa! (<u>bah</u>-heh-seh deh lah <u>meh</u>-sah)
Sit in the wheelchair!	¡Siéntese en la silla de ruedas! (syehn-teh-seh ehn lah sē̄ē-yah deh <u>rweh</u>-dahs)
Please get dressed!	¡Vístese usted, por favor! (<u>bē̄ēs</u>-teh-seh oos-tehd pawr fah-<u>bawr</u>)
Cross your legs!	¡Cruce las piernas! (<u>kroo</u>-seh lahs <u>pyehr</u>-nahs)
Don't be afraid!	¡No se asuste! (naw seh ah-<u>soos</u>-teh)
Come at 2:00 P. M. !	¡Venga a las dos de la tarde! (<u>behn</u>-gah ah lahs daws deh lah <u>tahr</u>-deh)
Take two tablets twice a day!	¡Tome dos pastillas dos veces al día! (taw-meh daws pahs-<u>tē̄ē</u>-yahs daws <u>beh</u>-sehs ahl <u>dē̄ē</u>-ah)
Do not have sexual relations for one month!	¡No tenga relaciones sexuales por un mes! (naw <u>tehn</u>-gah reh-lah-<u>syaw</u>-nehs sehg-<u>swah</u>-lehs pawr oon mehs)
Put two drops in each ear!	¡Ponga dos gotas en cada oreja! (<u>pawn</u>-gah daws <u>gaw</u>-tahs ehn <u>kah</u>-dah aw-<u>reh</u>-hah)
Swallow this pill!	¡Trague esta píldora! (<u>trah</u>-gheh <u>ehs</u>-tah <u>pē̄ēl</u>-daw-rah)
Swallow it!	¡Tráguela! (<u>trah</u>-gheh-lah)
Chew it!	¡Mastíquela! (mahs-<u>tē̄ē</u>-keh-lah)
Use hot (cold) compresses!	¡Usa compresas calientes (frías) (<u>oo</u>-sah kawm-<u>preh</u>-sahs kahl-<u>yehn</u>-tehs [<u>frē̄ē</u>-ahs])
Sit up!	¡Incorpórese! (<u>ē̄ēn</u>-kawr-<u>paw</u>-reh-seh)

Place yourself on a light diet.	Póngase a un régimen ligero. (pawn-gah-seh ah oon reh-hee-mehn lee-heh-raw)
Try to rest.	Trate de descansar. (trah-teh deh dehs-kahn-sahr)
Rinse your mouth!	¡Enjuáguese la boca! (ehn-hwah-gheh-seh lah baw-kah)
Give me your Blue Cross number!	¡Déme el número de su Cruz Azul! (deh-meh ehl noo-meh-raw deh soo kroos ah-sool)
- Medicare number	el numero de su Medicare (ehl noo-meh-raw deh soo Medicare)
- welfare card	tarjeta de ayuda social (tahr-heh-tah deh ah-yoo-dah saw-syahl)
- insurance policy number	el numero de su poliza de seguros (ehl noo-meh-raw deh soo paw-lee-sah deh seh-goo- raws)
Go into that room!	¡Váyese en ese cuarto! (bah-yeh-seh ehn eh-seh kwahr-taw)
Wait for me!	¡Espéreme! (ehs-peh-reh-meh)
Be careful!	¡Cuidado! (kwee-dah-daw)
Go to sleep!	¡Duérmese! (dwehr-meh-seh)
Don't speak!	¡No hable! (naw ah-bleh)
Eat!	¡Come! (kaw-meh)
Drink!	¡Beba! (beh-bah)
Relax!	¡Cálmese! (kahl-meh-seh)
Please repeat the question.	Tenga la bondad de repetir la pregunta. (tehn-gah lah bawn-dahd deh reh-peh-teer lah preh-goon-tah)
Walk!	¡Camine! (kah-mee-neh)
Stop!	¡Párese! (pah-reh-seh)
Show me your tongue!	¡Enséñeme la lengua! (ehn-sehn-yeh-meh lah lehn-gwah)
Take out your dentures!	¡Sáquese la dentadura! (sah-keh-seh lah dehn-tah-doo-rah)

Stretch your fingers!

¡Estire los dedos! (ehs-t$\overline{ee}$-reh laws deh-daws)

Use it exactly as the prescription indicates!

¡Úselo exactamente como le indica la prescripción! (oo-seh-law ehg-sahk-tah-mehn-teh kaw-maw leh $\overline{ee}$n-d$\overline{ee}$-kah lah preh-skr$\overline{ee}$p-syawn)

CCC

DISEASES AND INJURIES

DISEASES AND INJURIES	ENFERMEDADES Y HERIDAS (ehn-fehr-meh-dah-dehs ēē eh-rēē-dahs)
acne	acné (ahk-neh)
alcoholism	alcoholismo (ahl-kaw-aw-lēēs-maw)
allergy	alergia (ah-lehr-hyah)
amnesia	amnesia (ahm-neh-syah)
aneurysm	aneurisma (ah-neh-oo-rēēs-mah)
angina pectoris	angina del pecho (ahn-hēē-nah dehl peh-chaw)
apoplexy	apoplejía (ah-paw-pleh-hēē-ah)
appendicitis	apendicitis (ah-pehn-dēē-sēē-tees)
arteriosclerosis	arteriosclerosis (ahr-teh-ryaw-skleh-raw-sēēs)
arthritis	artritis (ahr-trēē-tēēs)
asphyxia	asfixia (ahs-fēēk-syah)
asthma	asma (ahz-mah)
attack	ataque (ah-tah-keh)
backache	dolor de espalda (daw-lawr deh ehs-pahl-dah)
blisters	ampollas (ahm-paw-yahs)
blood poisoning	envenenamiento de la sangre (ehn-beh-neh-nah-myehn-taw deh lah sahn-greh)
blood pressure	la presión de sangre (lah preh-syawn deh sahn-greh)
- high	alta (ahl-tah)
- low	baja (bah-hah)
bronchial asthma	asma bronquial (ahz-mah brawn-kyahl)
bronchitis	bronquitis (brawn-kēē-tēēs)
bruise	contusión (kawn-too-syawn)
burn	quemadura (keh-mah-doo-rah)

bursitis	bursitis (boor-$\overline{see}$-$\overline{tees}$)
cancer	cáncer (kahn-sehr)
chancre	chancro (chahn-kraw)
chicken pox	varicela (bah-$\overline{ree}$-seh-lah)
cholera	cólera (kaw-leh-rah)
chills	escalofríos (ehs-kah-law-$\overline{free}$-aws)
cirrhosis	cirrosis ($\overline{see}$-raw-$\overline{sees}$)
cold	catarro (kah-tah-raw)
colitis	colitis (kaw-$\overline{lee}$-$\overline{tees}$)
coma	coma (kaw-mah)
constipation	estreñimiento (ehs-trehn-y$\overline{ee}$-myehn-taw)
contusion	contusión (kawn-too-syawn)
convulsion	convulsiones (kawn-bool-syaw-nehs)
cough	tos (taws)
cramps	calambres (kah-lahm-brehs)
cyst	quiste ($\overline{kees}$-teh)
deafness	sordera (sawr-deh-rah)
diabetes	diabetes ($\overline{dee}$-ah-beh-tehs)
diarrhea	diarrea ($\overline{dee}$-ah-reh-ah)
diphtheria	difteria ($\overline{deef}$-teh-ryah)
dislocation	dislocación ($\overline{dees}$-law-kah-syawn)
dizziness	el vértigo (ehl vehr-t$\overline{ee}$-gaw)
dysentery	disentería (dee-sehn-teh-$\overline{ree}$-ah)
drug addiction	adicción a las drogas (ah-d$\overline{eek}$-syawn ah lahs draw-gahs)
earache	dolor de oídos (daw-lawr deh aw-$\overline{ee}$-daws)
eczema	eczema (ehk-seh-mah)
edema	edema (eh-deh-mah)
embolism	embolismo (ehm-baw-$\overline{leez}$-maw)

emphysema	enfisema (ehn-fee-seh-mah)
epilepsy	epilepsia (eh-pee-lehp-syah)
fatigue	fatiga (fah-tee-gah)
fainting	desmayo (dehs-mah-aw)
fever	fiebre (fyeh-breh)
fistula	fístula (fees-too-lah)
fracture	quebradura (keh-brah-doo-rah)
gallstones	cálculos en la vejiga (kahl-koo-laws ehn lah beh-hee-gah)
gangrene	gangrena (gahn-greh-nah)
gastritis	gastritis (gahs-tree-tees)
germ	germen (hehr-mehn)
glandular fever	fiebre glandular (fyeh-breh glahn-doo-lahr)
glaucoma	glaucoma (glah-oo-kaw-mah)
gonorrhea	gonorrea (gaw-naw-reh-ah)
goiter	bocio (baw-syaw)
grippe	gripe (gree-peh)
hay fever	fiebre del heno (fyeh-breh dehl eh-naw)
headache	dolor de cabeza (daw-lawr deh kah-beh-sah)
- migraine	jaqueca (hah-keh-kah)
heart failure	insuficiencia cardiaca (een-soo-fee-syehn-syah kahr-dyah-kah)
hemophilia	hemofilia (eh-maw-feel-yah)
hemorrhage	hemorragia (eh-maw-rah-hyah)
hemorrhoids	almorranas (ahl-maw-rah-nahs)
hepatitis	hepatitis (eh-pah-tee-tees)
hernia	hernia (ehr-nyah)
hoarseness	ronquera (rawn-keh-rah)
hypertension	hipertensión (ee-pehr-tehn-syawn)
hysteria	histeria (ees-teh-ryah)

indigestion	indigestión (een-dee-hehs-tyawn)
inflammation	inflamación (een-flah-mah-syawn)
influenza	influenza (een-floo-ehn-sah)
insanity	la locura (lah law-koo-rah)
insomnia	el insomnio (ehl een-sawm-nyaw)
intoxication	intoxicación (een-tawk-see-kah-syawn)
itch	picazón (pee-kah-sawn)
jaundice	ictericia (eek-teh-ree-syah)
kidney disease	enfermedad de riñones (ehn-fehr-meh-dahd deh reen-yaw-neh)
laryngitis	laringitis (lah-reen-hee-tees)
lesion	lesión (leh-syawn)
leukemia	leucemia (leh-oo-seh-myah)
malaria	malaria (mah-lah-ryah)
nausea	nausea (nah-oo-seh-ah)
neuralgia	neuralgia (neh-oo-rahl-hyah)
overweight	sobrepeso (saw-breh-peh-saw)
paralysis	parálisis (pah-rah-lee-sees)
Parkinson's disease	enfermedad Parkinson (ehn-fehr-meh-dahd pahr-keen-sawn)
peritonitis	peritonitis (peh-ree-taw-nee-tees)
phlebitis	flebitis (fleh-bee-tees)
phlegm	flema (fleh-mah)
pleuresy	pleuresía (pleh-oo-reh-see-ah)
pneumonia	pulmonía (pool-maw-nee-ah)
poliomyelitis	poliomielitis (paw-lyaw-myeh-lee-tees)
poisoning	envenenamiento (ehn-beh-neh-nah-myehn-taw)
prostration	postración (paws-trah-syawn)
psoriasis	soriasis (saw-ryah-sees)
pus	pus (poos)

pyorrhea	piorrea (pyaw-reh-ah)
rash	roncha (rawn-chah)
relapse	recaída (reh-kah-ee-dah)
rheumatic fever	fiebre reumática (fyeh-breh reh-oo mah-tee-kah)
rheumatism	reumatismo (reh-oo-mah-teez-maw)
rupture	hernia (ehr-nyah)
scab	postilla (paws-tee-yah)
scar	cicatriz (see-kah-trees)
scarlet fever	fiebre escarlatina (fyeh-breh ehs-kahr-lah-tee-nah)
sciatica	ciática (see-ah-tee-kah)
sinus congestion	congestión nasal (kawn-hehs-tyawn nah-sahl)
smallpox	viruela (bee-rweh-lah)
sore throat	dolor de garganta (daw-lawr deh gahr-gahn-tah)
sprain	torcedura (tawr-seh-doo-rah)
stomach ache	dolor de estómago (daw-lawr deh ehs-taw-mah-gaw)
stroke	ataque fulminante (ah-tah-keh fool-mee-nahn-teh)
sunstroke	insolación (een-saw-lah-syawn)
swelling	hinchazón (een-chah-sawn)
syphilis	sífilis (see-fee-lees)
tension	tensión (tehn-syawn)
tetanus	tétano (teh-tah-naw)
thrombosis, coronary	trombosis coronaria (trawm-baw-sees kaw-raw-nah-ryah)
tonsillitis	amigdalitis (ah-meeg-dah-lee-tees)
toothache	dolor de muelas (daw-lawr deh mweh-lahs)
tuberculosis	tuberculosis (too-behr-koo-law-sees)
tumor	tumor (too-mawr)

- benign	benigno (beh-n<u>ee</u>g-naw)
- malignant	maligno (mah-l<u>ee</u>g-naw)
typhoid fever	fiebre tifoidea (fyeh-breh t<u>ee</u>-f<u>awy</u>-dehah)
ulcer	úlcera (<u>ool</u>-seh-rah)
varicose veins	venas varicosas (<u>beh</u>-nahs bah-r<u>ee</u>-kaw-sahs)
venereal disease	enfermedad venérea (ehn-fehr-meh-<u>dahd</u> beh-neh-rey-ah)
vertigo	vértigo (<u>behr</u>-t<u>ee</u>-gaw)
virus	virus (b<u>ee</u>-roos)
vomit	vómito (<u>baw</u>-m<u>ee</u>-taw)
weakness	debilidad (deh-b<u>ee</u>-l<u>ee</u>-dahd)
wound	herida (eh-r<u>ee</u>-dah)

CBGB

SPECIALISTS IN MEDICINE

SPECIALISTS IN MEDICINE	ESPECIALISTAS EN MEDICINA (ehs-peh-syah-lees-tahs ehn meh-dee-see-nah)
anesthetist	anestesista (ah-nehs-teh-sees-tah)
bacteriologist	bacteriólogo (bahk-teh-ryaw-law-gaw)
cardiologist	cardiólogo (kahr-dyaw-law-gaw)
chiropodist	quiropedista (kee-raw-peh-dees-tah)
cytologist	citólogo (see-taw-law-gaw)
dermatologist	dermatólogo (dehr-mah-taw-law-gaw)
dentist	dentista (dehn-tees-tah)
dietician	dietista (dyeh-tees-tah)
doctor	médico (meh-dee-kaw)
gynecologist	ginecólogo (hee-neh-kaw-law-gaw)
neurologist	neurólogo (neh-oo-raw-law-gaw)
nurse	enfermera (ehn-fehr-meh-rah)
obstetrician	tocólogo (taw-kaw-law-gaw)
oculist	oculista (aw-koo-lees-tah)
pathologist	patólogo (pah-taw-law-gaw)
pediatrician	pediatra (peh-dyah-trah)
pharmacist	farmacéutico; boticario (fahr-mah-seh-oo-tee-kaw; baw-tee-kahr- yaw)
psychiatrist	psiquiatra (see-kyah-trah)
psychologist	psicólogo (see-kaw-law-gaw)

DISCHARGE AGAINST ADVICE OF DOCTOR OR HOSPITAL

If you care to leave against the advice of the hospital or of your own physician, you must sign this document that frees us from any liability.

I _____ , request that
      (name of patient, guardian, parent)

_____ be released and discharged from the
     (patient's name)

care of the _____ Hospital. I acknowledge that this departure request is against the advice of the doctor that is in charge of the/my case, and that the danger involved has been explained to me. I acknowledge that I have been advised to seek further medical care immediately.

I agree that _____ Hospital, all the officers and employees are free from liability for any injury, or after-effects that may result directly or indirectly by reason of this refusal of further hospitalization.

                            Signed _____

SALIDA CONTRA EL CONSEJO DEL MÉDICO O DEL HOSPITAL

Si quiere salir contra el consejo del hospital o de su propio médico, hay que firmar este documento que nos libra de toda responsabilidad.

Yo, _____, pido que
(nombre del paciente, el padre o el custodio)

a _____ se le despidan del cuidado del
(nombre del paciente)

hospital de _____. Me doy cuenta de que al salir contra el consejo del médico que está encargado del/de mi caso, hay cierto peligro que ya me lo han explicado. Yo reconozco que me han avisado que tenga que buscar más ciudado médico inmediatamente.

Estoy de acuerdo con el hecho de que el hospital de _____
su administración, y sus empleados, no tendrán ni culpa ni responsabilidad para cualquier daño o consecuencia que sucediera directamente o indirectamente por causa de este/mi rehuso de quedarme en el hospital.

Firma _____